Managing Menopause Naturally

with
Chinese Medicine

Honora Lee Wolfe

BLUE POPPY PRESS

Published by:
BLUE POPPY PRESS
A Division of Blue Poppy Enterprises, Inc.
5441 Western Ave., Suite 2
BOULDER, CO 80301

First Edition, November 1998
Second Printing, December, 2003
Third Printing, March, 2005
Fourth Printing, March, 2006

ISBN 0-936185-98-8

COMP Designation: Original work

Cover design by Eric Brearton
Blue Poppy Press

10 9 8 7 6 5 4

Printed at Fidlar Doubleday, Kalamazoo, MI on acid-free paper and soy inks

Other Books in this series include:
Curing Insomnia Naturally with Chinese Medicine
Curing Hay Fever Naturally with Chinese Medicine
Curing Headaches Naturally with Chinese Medicine
Better Breast Health Naturally with Chinese Medicine
Curing Depression Naturally with Chinese Medicine
Curing Arthritis Naturally with Chinese Medicine
Curing Fibromyalgia Naturally with Chinese Medicine
Curing PMS Naturally with Chinese Medicine
Curing IBS Naturally with Chinese Medicine
Controlling Diabetes Naturally with Chinese Medicine

Table of Contents

INTRODUCTION

Menopause is a popular topic these days. Magazine articles and books abound on the subject. As the first women of the Baby Boom generation approach and enter this passage, they are demanding more information, new and better options for medical treatment when necessary, and alternatives to standard Western medical therapies. Also, the women who are now in their 40s and 50s were and are some of the first movers and shakers of the women's movement in the 1960s and 70s. We are, as a group, quite vocal, and not likely to traverse any important passage in our lives without it being well documented.

Just having passed my 50th birthday, the subject of menopause comes often to my mind. As a practitioner of acupuncture, I see more and more women in the midst of this time in their lives. All those magazine articles, which 10 years ago I'd have barely skimmed if I'd have read them at all, seem to jump out of the table of contents and demand my attention. The impending loss of fertility and increasing reminders of aging in the mirror can no longer be ignored.

Whether or not we have come to terms with aging, mortality, or our existential dilemma, I and all my Baby Boom sisters must pass through menopause within the next decade or so. Typical of my generation, I want this coming life passage to be as free as possible from despair, confusion, loss of self-esteem, and physical discomfort. Of course I may not get my way, but my assumption is that other women have similar feelings, and it is because of this assumption that I add yet another to the list of books on menopause.

There are many fine books available on menopause and related topics, several of which I have listed in the Learning More section at the back. This book, however, is the only one (so far as I am aware) which discusses menopause entirely from the point of view of Traditional Chinese Medicine (TCM). It is my experience that TCM, its theories, and its various therapies have a great deal to offer the menopausal woman. This book is designed to help women understand the theories of TCM *vis-à-vis* menopause, and to decide if TCM may help ease the possible physical and emotional discomforts which too often attend it.

Secondly, this book is about the prevention of the symptoms of what is called menopausal syndrome. Offered herein are a number of self-help ideas and disciplines to reduce stress, create purpose and self-esteem, and improve quality of life during menopause, or at any other time which is emotionally or physically trying.

Finally, this book is my own attempt to come to terms with approaching menopause and aging, and to document and share a part of that process with my readers. I wish us all good luck and good health.

THE WESTERN MEDICAL DESCRIPTION OF
MENOPAUSE & MENOPAUSAL SYNDROME

According to modern Western medicine, natural menopause is described as the transitional phase of a woman's life when menstrual function ceases due to age-related declining ovarian function usually occurring between the ages of 40 and 50. Around the end of the fourth or beginning of the fifth decade of life, a woman's ovaries cease producing estrogen and progesterone despite hormonal stimulation from the pituitary gland. Ovulation becomes less and less frequent and eventually stops. Estrogen blood levels fall below the point necessary to produce uterine bleeding so that periods slowly cease. Estrogen levels continue to decline slowly over another year or so until no estrogen at all is secreted from the ovaries.

It seems that it takes a while for the pituitary to get the message that the ovaries are no longer functioning. It continues to produce follicle stimulating hormone (FSH) and luteinizing hormone (LH) at high levels to try to get the ovaries to respond. The levels of these two hormones in the bloodstream becomes elevated at the time of menopause, while estrogen and progesterone levels are falling.

Although no longer secreted by the ovaries, estrogen is still being produced in the body, but in a slightly different form called estrone. It is manufactured by the body's fat cells from a precursor hormone called androstenedione, which is largely produced by the adrenal glands. This is one possible reason why

3

some menopausal women put on weight, in the body's attempt to produce enough estrogen.[1]

According to Western medicine, early or premature menopause, or menopause prior to age 40, may occur for a variety of reasons. The most common of these include response to viral infection, inherited chromosomal abnormality, defects in gonadotropin secretion, autoimmune disorders, enzymatic defects, excessive smoking, or cancerous growths.[2]

Artificial menopause automatically follows the surgical removal of the ovaries, irradiation of the ovaries, or radium implants in the uterus, thus destroying them and their ability to secrete estrogen.[3]

Although the transition of menopause may occur without symptoms, at least 75% of women experience the most common menopausal symptoms—hot flashes.[4] According to modern Western medicine, these are due to instability of the brain's relay system, its neurotransmitters, which are affected by the lowered levels of estrogen in the blood stream as menopause progresses. This instability affects our autonomic nervous system (ANS). It is the ANS which is responsible for our body's thermostatic control, contraction and dilation of the blood vessels and skin pores,

---

[1] Lyttleton, Jane, "Topics in Gynaecology Part One: Menopause", *Journal of Chinese Medicine*, Sussex, UK, #33, May, 1990, p. 5

[2] Berkow, Robert, and Fletcher, Andrew, *The Merck Manual oa Diagnosis and Therapy*, 15th Edition, Merck, Sharp, & Dohme Research Laboratories, Rahway, NJ, 1987, p. 1697

[3] Ibid., p. 1713

[4] McVeigh, Gloria, "Mastering Menopause: A Plan of Action for Every Symptom and Side Effect", *Prevention Magazine*, Vol. 42, #4, April, 1990, p. 48

perspiration, and other automatic physiological responses of our body. Another way to think about the ANS is that it is responsible for all the many things which go on in our bodies which are not usually within our conscious control.

It can take awhile for this brain relay system to readjust itself to a new level of blood estrogen. For the average woman this usually means about a year of hot flashes, although some women experience them for much shorter or longer periods of time and some not at all.

A related problem is night sweats, which are related to hot flashes, but experienced at night and often involve a complete drenching of one's bed clothes and feelings of being chilled instead of being overheated. These are often more problematic than hot flashes because they disturb a woman's sleep, thereby causing other kinds of problems. In fact, some sources feel that the fatigue, irritability, and insomnia which some menopausal women report are merely side effects of frequent night sweat episodes.[5]

Another common symptom of menopause is irregular periods with extremely heavy bleeding. Again, this seems to be related to the erratic brain relay system and lack of ovulation which results in irregular levels of estrogen in relationship to progesterone. Fibroid tumors, endometriosis, and uterine cancer are also possible causes. Excessive stress can make this problem worse. Excessive menopausal or postmenopausal bleeding is usually treated with estrogen replacement therapy (ERT), birth control pills, D&C, or, in extreme cases, hysterectomy.

Other symptoms which can effect women during menopause include depression, palpitations, numbness and tingling in the

---

[5] Ibid., p. 48

limbs, urinary frequency or incontinence, back pain, vaginal dryness or irritation, and various gastrointestinal disorders.[6]

Sometimes Western medical practitioners will look for an organic dysfunction responsible for these difficulties, such as high blood pressure and thyroid or pituitary disorders. Most often, however, the medical texts counsel the doctor to try and evaluate how many of these symptoms are psychogenic in origin.[7] In other words, modern Western medicine often tends to dismiss some aspects of menopausal syndrome as psychological or emotionally induced. While there is no doubt that psychoemotional factors play a role in many modern women's health problems, this attitude on the part of Western practitioners may also be because Western medicine posits no clear etiology or cause for many of these signs and symptoms other than estrogen deficiency.

Because Western medicine essentially defines menopausal problems as a lack of estrogen production, the main Western therapy prescribed for menopausal women is estrogen replacement therapy (ERT). The pros and cons of ERT are discussed in Chapter 11 of this book as well as in many other books on menopause. While not a panacea for the symptoms of aging, ERT can diminish or eliminate many of the troublesome symptoms of menopausal syndrome at least for a while. Especially hot flashes, night sweats, and joint or back pain due to bone decalcification are often positively affected by ERT. ERT also seems to have a positive effect on the elasticity of the arteries, thereby reducing the risk of heart disease.[8] Estrogen creams are also used

---

[6] Berkow, R., and Fletcher, A., op.cit., p. 1713

[7] Ibid., p. 1714

[8] Gambrell Jr., Don R., *Estrogen Replacement Therapy*, Second Edition, Essential Medical Information Systems, Inc., Dallas, TX, 1990, p. 29

locally to reverse vaginal inflammation and sensitivity as well as some cases of urinary incontinence.

ERT therapy, however, does have risks. It has been implicated as a factor in certain types of breast cancer. It is also linked to higher rates of endometrial cancer (cancer of the uterine lining). However, preliminary research indicates that the use of lower doses of estrogen with progesterone added for part of the month reduce or negate this latter risk.[9] Additionally, ERT is usually not prescribed for women who smoke due to the possible increased risk in these women for blood clots and stroke, or for women with gallbladder disease. Finally, some women will have to discontinue ERT due to excess vaginal bleeding, sore breasts, nausea and vomiting, uterine cramps, or abdominal bloating. [10]

Other therapies which are sometimes prescribed for menopausal women can include androgens or male sex hormones for loss of sexual desire, thyroid hormones for boosting energy, antidepressants for severe depression, psychotherapy and mild sedatives for irritability, anxiety, or sleep disturbances, and large doses of calcium to protect against progressive osteoporosis. Biofeedback therapy is sometimes recommended to help regulate and control ANS responses for improving hot flash symptoms.

Other problems may occur after menopause including postmenopausal bleeding, serious bone decalcification (osteoporosis), and increased incidence of heart disease. These problems will be discussed later in the sections on Chinese medical theories relating to menopause, preventive therapies professional treatments, and in chapters 11 and12.

---

[9] Greenwood, Sadja, *Menopause Naturally, Preparing for the Second Half of Life*, Revised Edition, Volcano Press, Volcano, CA, 1989, p. 86

[10] Gambrell, Jr., Don R., *op.cit.*, p. 11

I have not gone into great detail about Western medicine and menopausal syndrome. This is because Western medicine offers only a few satisfactory treatments for menopausal syndrome. Traditional Chinese Medicine (TCM), on the other hand, has many safe and effective treatments for menopausal complaints and much wisdom concerning the whys and wherefores of these complaints. It is this information that I would like to share with American women. There are many good books available which do discuss Western medicine and menopausal physiology quite completely. I refer the reader to these for more detail in the area of Western medicine and its research or knowledge on the subject of menopause. (See the Learning More section in the back of this book.)

WHY CHOOSE TRADITIONAL CHINESE MEDICINE?

Chinese medicine has at least 2000 years of recorded clinical history and within that time many styles of medical practice have been developed. Since the Chinese communist revolution in 1949 the government of China has supported one particular style of Chinese medicine, which is called Traditional Chinese Medicine (TCM). In the last two decades, many Westerners have gone to China to study TCM, and it has become the dominant style of Chinese medicine taught and practiced in the U.S. with over 25 schools, a national school accrediting body, and a national board examination to test for minimum competency. Practitioners of TCM in the U.S. may have training in acupuncture, herbal medicine, massage, and/or a few other related modalities. When I use the term Chinese medicine in this book, I am referring to TCM.

There are many reasons why TCM is a good choice for women with gynecological problems, menopausal syndrome included. I'll try to outline them as succinctly as possible.

Chinese Medicine Is Holistic

First, Chinese medicine is one of the most holistic medical systems available today. This can be seen in a number of ways. One example is that it does not segment health problems as either physical or psychological entities. One of the most enlightened aspects of Chinese medicine is that it never created a mind/body dualism. To think that one does not affect the other is absurd. To a practitioner of TCM, an emotional or mental event or experience

9

is only another piece of diagnostic information, no different or less important that a physical sign or symptom. Treatment plans using acupuncture or herbal medicine typically include certain emotional tendencies or experiences as part of the overall pattern of disharmony being treated. While some practitioners of Chinese medicine may suggest the support of psychotherapy, just as many others may feel that acupuncture treatment is often as effective a method of working with certain emotional states. Classically, Chinese medical theory expects specific mental/emotional conditions to go along with certain disease patterns, and expects these emotional symptoms to respond to treatment as well as any physical symptom.

Further, in Chinese medicine each and every sign and symptom is only understood or interpreted in relationship to all the others. For example, a woman may come to a practitioner with complaints such as lower abdominal gas and bloating, loose bowel movements, appetite fluctuations, premenstrual symptoms such as irritability and breast tenderness, dizziness, fatigue, and low back pain. The Western medical practitioner might prescribe one medicine for the loose bowels, another for the appetite fluctuations, another for the PMS irritability, another for the back pain, and yet another for the dizziness. Furthermore, the MD might choose to send the patient to two or three specialists — an internist or gastroenterologist for the digestive problems, a gynecologist for the PMS symptoms, an orthopedist for the back pain, and a neurologist for the dizziness.

On the other hand, a good practitioner of Traditional Chinese Medicine sees and understands the *whole pattern* of this patient as if she were a landscape painting with various aspects — water, trees, mountains, etc. — but all of one piece. The practitioner then prescribes singly or a combination of acupuncture, herbal, nutritional, exercise, and/or massage therapies to work effectively with the entire pattern that each patient presents. Done skillfully, Chinese medicine need not, indeed cannot, separate a person into segmented parts treating one symptom or part at the expense of another. Each part is only relevant in relationship to the whole of each patient's personal "landscape". Further, any change of even one sign or symptom may change the entire pattern, and therefore the entire treatment plan. In this way Traditional Chinese Medicine is indeed a holistic and humane system of medicine.

Chinese Medicine Is Individualized

The second reason why a person might consider the use of Chinese medicine is that, because of its holistic view, it is more specific for each patient's needs than is Western medicine. A good example of this is the treatment of the Western named disease diabetes. The basic Western prescription for diabetes is insulin, which comes in several forms. These largely work on the principle of preventing hyperglycemia and glucosuria (elevated sugar in the blood and urine). This in turn helps minimize the damage to blood vessels and nervous tissue associated with severe cases of diabetes, and prevents insulin shock.[11] In Chinese medicine, however, a person with a Western diagnosis of diabetes must still go through a complete TCM diagnosis. This diagnosis can reveal any one of five or six simple patterns and a myriad of individualized complex patterns of disharmony which can account for a specific person's diabetes. Each of these patterns requires a different kind of treatment from the others, making it more specific to that particular person's needs and imbalance. Such personally tailored treatment lessens the possibility of that person experiencing unnecessary side effects.

---

[11] Berkow, R., and Fletcher, A., *op.cit.*, p. 1075

11

Chinese Medicine Has No Side Effects

The third reason for choosing Traditional Chinese Medicine is that it is noniatrogenic. That is to say, if the diagnosis has been correct, the treatments prescribed by Chinese medicine have no side effects. Although some side effects initially may be experienced with herbal medicines, they are usually mild, and can be corrected by adjustments in the herbal formula. Acupuncture rarely has unwanted side effects. Occasionally a client will report being excessively drowsy for a few hours after a treatment, or mild numbness or aching at one or another site of needle insertion, but long term or debilitating side effects are unknown. Even if the desired therapeutic effect *vis à vis* the major complaint is not achieved, most patients report feeling relaxed and comfortable after a treatment. For most people seeking Chinese medical help no negative side effects are experienced. In contradistinction, most drugs listed in a *Physician's Desk Reference (PDR)* have at least some expected and normal side effects and many have potentially serious irreversible ones.

Chinese Medicine Is Preventive Medicine

Another reason why TCM is a good choice for women is because it is energetic medicine as well as or even more than material medicine. To understand the importance of this we must again use a comparison to Western medicine. Western medical science is based on a reductionist material model of reality. This means that Western medicine mostly understands disease mechanisms by identifying and measuring smaller and smaller particles of matter and then manipulating those particles through drug therapy or removing sections of matter from within the body. Treatment can only be given if there is a measurable or quantifiable change in some bodily tissue or substance. This means Western medical treatment can be given only after disease has already progressed to the point of creating a quantifiable material change in the body.

Chinese medicine, by contrast, is energetic and functional in its orientation. The theories of Chinese medicine show us that often before any *measurable* change can occur in the tissues of the body, there will be energetic or functional changes which the patient will experience subjectively. Persons may complain of having a lump in the throat or sighing all the time, of feeling inappropriate anger or feeling that their lower body is cold as ice, or that they have feeling of anxious emptiness in their heart. To the Western MD, none of these symptoms may be clinically useful, yet blood or other tissue samples may also reveal nothing of clinical value. The person may have what Western medicine calls a purely functional disorder. The patient may clearly feel diseased, but the Western doctor may not be able to make a diagnosis. To the practitioner of TCM, however, these types of symptoms have great clinical meaning. They indicate to him or her that energetic changes have occurred in the body/mind which, if untreated over a period of time, will lead to tissue changes, and therefore more serious diseases.

This is significant because it means that a good practitioner of TCM can treat disease at a more fundamental level which then helps prevent the onset of more serious disease. Therefore, Chinese medicine is good preventive medicine, as well as being able to treat signs and symptoms which Western medicine sees as subclinical and therefore does not recognize as disease. This is especially important in the treatment of gynecological disorders, so many of which involve functional, emotional, and from the Western medical point of view, often subclinical signs and symptoms.

Chinese Medicine's History of Success

Traditional Chinese Medicine has a long history of clinical success. The literature recording and verifying this history extends back over 2000 years or more and includes over 30,000 volumes. By comparison, modern Western medicine as it has been practiced over the last 50-100 years is a very young system. Many of the newest Western medical treatments for a given ailment have yet to be tried over even one generation allowing determination or measurement of long term side effects. On the other hand, many Western medical treatments are quite wonderful and it is not my intention to say that we should dismiss the system out of hand. Rather modern Western medicine might be best seen as part of a larger system of medicine which allows people more options, and more levels of response. At times the swift and heroic treatments of Western medicine are useful and necessary in serious, acute, or life-threatening situations. For chronic or functional disorders, however, Chinese medicine offers a viable alternative, indeed an effective and humane alternative in areas which Western medicine offers few options or only treatments with many uncomfortable and possibly dangerous side effects.

Chinese Medicine Offers Self-Empowerment

Gynecology in general is an area in which Chinese medicine shines. Its treatment is humane, without side effects, and relatively inexpensive for a wide variety of disorders. Further-more, Chinese medical theories are based upon direct observation of nature, as opposed to the abstract, mathematical complexities of histology and biochemistry in Western medicine. It is easier for a patient to grasp an understanding of their disease and its process as seen and described by Chinese medical theory, and it is usually far more empowering. To tell a patient, for example, that she has abnormally shaped red blood cells, or an elevated white blood cell count suggesting the presence of a bacterial infection, which is treated by so many days or weeks of this or that drug, may not be meaningful and may not allow her an understanding or an entrance for working with her disorder herself.[12] On the other hand, a practitioner of TCM may, for example, tell a patient that her liver and stomach are overheated. This is due to congested energy rather like heat in a pressure cooker. This condition, the practitioner continues, is related largely to dietary factors and stress, and these can be controlled by limiting certain foods in the diet, and by controlling stress which is like turning off the fire underneath the pressure cooker. Acupuncture may help reroute the heat or clear it from the organs which it is affecting. Such patient education gives the client a metaphor for seeing her psychophysical process, logically leading to possible responses she can make to improve or control her own health. In this way Chinese medicine is immediately understandable and empowering for the client. Its explanations and metaphors describing the disease process come from the natural world, to which most people can easily relate. It is not conceptually distant and opaque.

To recapitulate, there are six reasons why a woman may want to consider Chinese medical treatment for a menopausal, or any other gynecological disorder:

1. It is holistic, describing and evaluating the whole landscape of the body/mind, each part and piece in relationship to the others.

2. As a medical system, it has no inherently dangerous or trouble-some side effects.

---

[12] I feel that more MD's are trying to provide their clients with information, both written and verbal, at a level which they can understand and which gives the client more personal power in their own healing process.

3. Its diagnostic techniques allow for great precision in seeing each individual quite specifically and thereby creating treatment plans which are equally precise.

4. It is a medicine which is more effective at manipulating energy than matter, and sees energetic change in the body as more fundamental than material change. By treating energetic imbalance effectively, gross material or substantial disease need not arise. This means that Chinese medicine is a preventive system of medicine.

5. Chinese medicine has a long, clinically verified history of effective treatment for most types of disease, including gynecology.

6. It is an understandable and empowering system of medicine, allowing patients a chance to understand their disease process and thereby the chance to participate in their healing process.

CHINESE MEDICAL THEORIES
PERTAINING TO MENOPAUSE

In order to understand the phenomenon of menopause from the point of view of Traditional Chinese Medicine (TCM), we first must understand the theories explaining menstruation, organ function, the emotions in relationship to the organs, yin and yang, and the production, storage and circulation of blood, energy (*qi*), body fluids, and vital essence (*jing*). In this chapter we will try to break down these theories into simple parts which, when put back together, will allow the reader to understand what a doctor of TCM understands when he or she evaluates a patient with menopausal symptoms.

The Map Is Not the Terrain

For the reader to understand these theories, she must, as much as possible, forget about Western medical science, biology, and physiology. Chinese medicine has its own complete and self-contained description of the body and its functions. Its theories of physiology cannot and should not be compared with Western medicine. I like to use the metaphor of different kinds of maps. There are rainfall maps, population maps, topographic maps, and road maps. Each is self-contained and logical according to its own criteria. Each is a description of one aspect of reality and each has a different use. This is also true of Chinese medicine and Western medicine. Each has its own logic, rationale, and self-consistent view of reality. But each is only one map - and the map is not the terrain. In our culture, Western medical science has come to be believed as somehow really REAL, instead of one possible view, one level of how things are. Neither view negates the other, but it is best not to try and mix or cross reference one to the other.

Another challenge in understanding Chinese medicine has to do with translation. Our language is linear, deductive, and denotative. Chinese is elliptical, inductive, and connotative. Yet we must use certain words to translate from the Chinese. In this book the most important words presenting translational difficulty have to do with body organs and tissues. The word blood is a good example of this problem. In Chinese medicine the blood *(xue)* means something more than just the red fluid which flows through the arteries and veins. It has to do with the function of nutrition and nurturance altogether. It is energetic as well as substantive. Therefore, once again, the reader must forget her notions of blood from the point of view of Western physiology in order to understand the Chinese concept of blood.

This is also true for the various Chinese organs, whose descriptions sometimes overlap with those of Western physiology, but are much broader, and conceptually quite different. Chinese organs are described by energetic, not chemical, functions, and must be thought of as freshly as possible in the reader's mind. Unfortunately, we have no adequate words to use in our language and so must use the words we have. However, unless a word is noted as being specifically a Western medical term, the reader must set aside her old concepts of that word, and try as best she can to adopt a beginner's mind, allowing a new map of the body to come into focus.

A Word About Yin and Yang

Yin and yang are terms in Chinese philosophy and medicine used to describe the polarization of all phenomena in the universe. As such, a basic understanding of yin and yang is vital to understanding Chinese medicine. As a result of the constant flux and interplay of these two opposing forces, all things evolve and devolve.

In the West, these words have been bandied about in many erroneous ways, and there are many misconceptions as to their meaning. Let us try to present them as clearly as possible in relation to the body and to Chinese medicine.

1. Yin and yang are generic concepts describing opposing aspects or phenomena in nature. They may represent any two opposing objects or concepts or opposite aspects within a single object.

2. In all situations, yin and yang are interdependent. One does not, cannot exist without the other, just as dark implies light. In opposition they create unity.

3. Their relationship is in constant flux within a living being or system, just as the seasons follow one upon the next. Although health is the relative balance of yin and yang, this is never a static balance.

4. In the human body or in nature, two natural symbols guide the classification of all other phenomena into yin and yang categories. These are fire and water. Fire is yang and water is yin. Any object that has properties or causes energetic change similar to those of fire or water may be described similarly as predominately yang or yin.

5. Yin and yang are only relative concepts. An object or phenomenon can be yin in one situation or comparison, and yang in another. They are not absolute; they imply no value judgment.

6. Within the body it is said that qi (movement and function) is yang in relation to blood (substance and nourishment) and that

essence (primal substance) is yin in relationship to spirit (primal movement). Within the body yin and yang must remain in dynamic harmonious balance. Yang must quicken yin; yin must nourish, cool, and root yang. Life requires them both, as the seed sprouts in spring only with the nourishment of the soil and melting snow (yin), and the warmth of the sun (yang).

7. If the harmonious relationship of interpromotion and restraint is lost between yin and yang in the body or in nature, disorder and discomfort will arise. Again, this will be explained in greater detail in later chapters. The chart below gives some basic opposite aspects of physiology in relationship to yin and yang.

However, in looking at this chart, it is of utmost importance to remember that these yin/yang dichotomies only describe the relationships between these givens. Darkness is yin only in comparison to light. It in no way implies that females are dark or males are light or that females are cold and males are hot. Nothing is inherently yin or yang. Something is more yin or yang in relationship to something else. Ultimately, there is no thing that is yin or yang. Yin/yang theory is only a description of one thing in relationship to another.

Yang	**Yin**
Heaven	Earth
Day	Night
Spring/Summer	Autumn/Winter
Male	Female
Hot	Cold
Light	Darkness
Light	Heavy
Upward/Outward	Downward/Inward
Surface	Bones
Bowels	Organs
Agitated	Calm

Vital Substances: Qi, Blood, Body Fluids & Essence

As stated above, Chinese medical physiology is quite different from Western physiology, and volumes have been written on it. Although such detail is not necessary in this case, a minimal understanding of a few key words and concepts will be helpful to the reader. Four of the most important of these are qi, blood, body fluids, and essence. These words are difficult if not impossible to translate, but we can get a basic idea by considering their functions.

Qi

This is perhaps the most difficult of these four words to describe. One English language writer has called qi "energy on the verge of becoming matter, or matter on the verge of becoming energy."[13] Dr. Liang, director of one of the first colleges of acupuncture in the U.S. describes qi as follows:

> The concept of qi is unlimited. Any movement, regardless of how small or how large, how brief or how long, how quick or how slow is caused by qi. When qi concentrates it is called matter, and where it spreads it is called space. When qi gathers together it is called life, and when it separates it is called death. When qi flows it is called health and when it is blocked there is disease.
>
> Planets depend upon it for their brightness. Weather is formed by it. The seasons are caused by it. Man cannot stand outside

---

[13] Kaptchuk, Ted, *The Web That Has No Weaver*, Congdon & Weed, NY, 1983, p. 35-36

of qi. It supports him and permeates him as water is contained within the ocean. [14]

These are eloquent and poetic descriptions, which give some idea of the difficulty of translating so many Chinese medical terms. The simplest way to understand qi, however, is that qi is function (as compared to structure). It is yang in relationship to blood being yin. In the body, all physiologic activity is described by and dependent upon the movements and mutations of qi. The five basic functions or intrinsic characteristics of qi are:

Propulsion/movement: Qi propels the blood, transports nutritive substance to the entire body, and circulates the body fluids.

Warming: Qi maintains the body temperature and by its warming nature energizes all the functional activities of the organism.

Defense: Qi defends the body surface against invasion by exogenous pathogens.

Transformation: Qi transforms the blood and body fluids. It creates these out of the raw materials derived from respiration and digestion.

Restraint or Astringency: The qi holds the blood within its vessels, the body fluids within the body, and the organs up against gravity.

We will see later what happens when there is any breakdown in any of these functions.

---

[14] Dr. Liang, as quoted in course notes, Dechen Yonten Dzo Institute of Buddhist Medicine, Feb., 1986

Blood (*Xue*)

Described as the substance which flows through the vessels, the main function of blood is to nourish. It is more material, physical, or yin than qi. In the *Nei Jing Su Wen (Inner Classic Simple Questions)*, one of Chinese medicine's first classics, it is said that "The qi commands the blood, the blood is the mother of the qi." This statement describes the basic difference between qi and blood or the yin/yang polarity between them. If qi is responsible for movement, warmth, transformation, and restraint of the blood, blood is the underlying nourishment which fuels these functions of qi. Without blood or nourishment (yin), the qi (yang) has no root, no material or substantial foundation or mother. Without qi (yang) to move, warm, and transform the blood (yin), the blood is inert, without force or direction. As always yin and yang are completely interdependent.

Another statement from the *Nei Jing Su Wen* elucidates the function of blood for us more fully.

> When the liver receives blood, the eyes can see. When the legs receive blood, they are able to walk. When the hands receive blood, they are able to grip. When the fingers receive blood, they are able to grasp.

The blood is the nutritive substance which the qi then consumes and transforms to create function.

Blood also has a strong relationship to healthy psychological functioning which will be discussed in the section covering organ functions and emotions. When there is adequate blood to nourish each organ, a person's emotions/spirit will be calm.

Body Fluids

Also a part of the yin of the body, body fluids are a general term for all normal water/fluids within the body. They themselves are also subdivided into yin and yang. The yin are those thick viscous fluids which nourish the joints and internal organs and which cushion the brain and spinal cord. The yang are the lighter, thinner fluids, such as tears, saliva, sweat, urine, gastric juice, and interstitial fluid. The functions of the body fluids are to moisten the skin, hair, joints, organs, and tissues of the body, and to facilitate smooth movement of joints and other body parts. Blood and body fluids are derived from a common source and may affect each other. For instance, consumption of blood may injure the body fluids and vice versa.

It is the qi which is responsible for the movement and transformation of body fluids. Qi moves and transports the body fluids to all parts of the body. Therefore, an insufficiency of qi may result in body fluids accumulating somewhere in the body as pathologic dampness.

Essence

Essence refers to the vital physical essence of the body, its seminal basis. It is the primary substantial element responsible for determining physical growth and development and maintenance of life activity and metabolism. It is the most primal stuff from which our being unfolds. The outward physical manifestation of essence in women is (menstrual) blood; in men it is semen. It is the material base necessary for the creation of a new being, the creation of life. Therefore essence is yin in relationship to spirit, which is the nonmaterial or yang impetus necessary for the creation of life. As we will see below, in Chinese

24

medicine there are two types of essence, pre and postnatal. The relationship of essence to qi and blood is somewhat complex, and due to its importance in relationship to menopause, this relationship deserves a section of its own.

Essence, Qi, Blood & Aging

When a baby is conceived, it is endowed with a certain complement of essence from its parents based upon their constitutional vigor, age, and current health. This is called in Chinese medicine prenatal essence. This is one's constitutional inheritance and it cannot be augmented. When this supply is used up in the process of living, a person dies, very much like a candle which goes out when its wax is used up. This fact is central to understanding the importance of menopause as a homeostatic mechanism which slows down the aging process in women.

When a baby is born, it takes its first breath and suckles its first food. From that moment on it is responsible for the creation of its own qi and blood, which previously it received from its mother in utero. This is called the postnatal production of qi and blood. When a person is young and healthy and their digestion strong, they typically produce an overabundance of qi and blood or more than their body needs to function and maintain health day to day. During sleep each night this surplus is transformed by the body into postnatal or acquired essence. This is stored by the kidneys, as if in a bank, for use in emergencies or if the production of postnatal essence falls off for any reason. As long as digestion is good and the body is not overtaxed or ill, there will be surplus production of postnatal qi and blood and, therefore, abundant postnatal or acquired essence. This postnatal essence bolsters prenatal essence and slows down the consumption of that original endowment. It is rather like living on the interest from one's wise investments (good diet and healthy lifestyle producing plenty of qi and blood) so that one does not consume one's initial capital (their prenatal essence).

In women this surplus of qi and blood which leads to production of postnatal or acquired essence is directly related to the menses. From the point of view of Chinese medicine, menstruation is due to a superabundance of blood produced by a healthy woman which brims over about every 28 days.

At around the age of 35-40, this production cycle begins to slow down with the natural process of aging. The digestion becomes less efficient, therefore producing less qi and blood. This is relevant to menopause for two interrelated reasons. First, it means that, over time, there is not the production of the super-abundance of blood required for menstruation. Second, it means that less postnatal or acquired essence is available to supplement prenatal essence. This leads to the consumption of prenatal essence which describes the aging process.

One of the reasons why menopause is a necessary, vital homeo-static mechanism in women's bodies is that by ending the monthly loss of blood, the consumption of both blood and prenatal essence is slowed down. This is because, as it is said in the classics, essence and blood share a common source, the kidneys. When blood is lost with the menses each month, some essence is also lost, since the menstrual blood, as stated above, is the physical manifestation of essence in women. As the body metabolism slows down and less blood, qi, and postnatal essence is created, the body can ill-afford the monthly loss of blood (and essence) of menstruation. The body's wisdom slows and then stops the menstrual flow, allowing the body to hold onto the blood and essence, which are now more pre-cious since less is being created.

Thus, the menopause allows a woman the possibility for another 20 to 30 years of relative good health, with much slower decline than would be the case if menstruation continued. Menopause, while itself a sign of aging, actually slows down the aging process by preventing the unnecessary loss of blood and essence. Figure 1 below gives a visual overview of the processes we have just gone over.

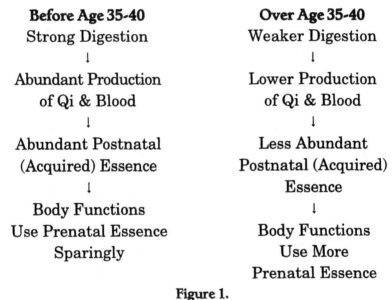

Before Age 35-40
Strong Digestion
↓
Abundant Production
of Qi & Blood
↓
Abundant Postnatal
(Acquired) Essence
↓
Body Functions
Use Prenatal Essence
Sparingly

Over Age 35-40
Weaker Digestion
↓
Lower Production
of Qi & Blood
↓
Less Abundant
Postnatal (Acquired)
Essence
↓
Body Functions
Use More
Prenatal Essence

Figure 1.
The Creation of Qi, Blood, and Essence In Relationship To Aging

Viscera, Channels, and the Seven Emotions

Chinese medicine recognizes five yin viscera and six yang bowels in the body. As stated in the introduction to this chapter, while there is some overlapping, the Chinese descriptions of these viscera and bowels are very different from those of Western medical physiology. These differences are largely due to the fact

27

that all descriptions of anything in TCM are energetic more than material. Chinese medicine is not much concerned with the chemical composition of cells or tissues within the organs, or even with the gross physical structure of the organs. Rather its emphasis is on what functions or energetic transformations in the body an organ engenders, controls, promotes, or inhibits, and what happens or doesn't happen when an organ is imbalanced or diseased. Because I want to emphasize to the reader that the Chinese organs of the same English name are not the same as what we all learned in high school biology, I refer to these Chinese concepts as viscera (single: viscus).

In addition to being responsible for various internal transformations resulting in the creation and/or storage and release of pure substances (qi, blood, body fluids, essence), each viscus is also responsible for the normal functioning of a particular layer of body tissue, a particular sensory ability, one of the five "spirits" or aspects of the psyche, and the expression of a particular emotion. (See Figure 2). This means that a Chinese organ is not just a piece of differentiated tissue within the abdominal or thoracic cavity, but is a functional orb or a zone of greatly concentrated energetic activity within the overall energetic grid or circuitry of the body. Each organ is an energy vortex and the sphere of influence of each organ can and does extend to many other parts of the body, via pathways which Chinese medicine calls channels and network vessels.

Viscus	Tissue	Sense	Emotion
Heart	Blood vessels	Speech	Joy/Fright
Spleen	Muscles & flesh	Taste	Excessive Thinking/Worry
Lung	Skin/ Body Hair	Smell	Grief
Kidneys	Bones/ Head Hair	Hearing	Fear
Liver	Sinews	Sight	Anger

Figure 2.
Chinese Viscera's Areas of Influence

Channels and network vessels, or what are more commonly referred to in the English language literature as meridians, are sometimes described by Western authors as the electrical wiring of the body. They are the pathways over which the qi flows, the routes by which the viscera and the various types of qi manifest their functions and communicate with each other. These channels and network vessels are not visible conduits which can be seen upon dissection of the body, but their existence can be measured electrically and can also be felt by the propagation of acupuncture needle sensation along their pathways. The pathways of these channels are quite distinct and have been well delineated in the Chinese medical literature for over two millennia. Current research suggests that these channels over which the qi flows are the fascial planes in the connective tissue which bind the entire body together into one energetically connected unit.

Each viscus and bowel has its own related channel, but the channel and network system as a whole forms one interconnected grid which functions as a sophisticated communication system. It is not within the scope of this book to describe in detail all the pathways of each viscus's channel or how they interrelate, but in our discussion of specific symptoms in the following chapter, we will refer to certain channel routes to describe why certain symptoms appear in specific parts of the body. Readers interested in learning more about the channels and network vessels are referred to the Suggested Reading section in the back for books on Chinese medicine which contain detailed descriptions of this transportation and communication system.

As stated above, each viscus is related to, or facilitates the expression of one or more emotions. The experience of any emotion is, from the Chinese medical point of view, merely the subjective experience of qi flowing in specific directions. For example, fear is the emotion which corresponds to the kidneys. The kidney qi normally moves downward to more the urine out of the body. In moments of great fear, the kidney qi sinks or moves rapidly down. The physical experience of this sinking may be great urgency to urinate or defecate or a literal sinking feeling in the body as the kidney qi moves down.

Normally, an emotion comes or "bubbles up" as it were, is experienced, and passes on based upon the organism's reaction to an appropriate stimuli. This is the normal, healthy experience of emotional states. If life situations cause one particular emotion to arise continually or to remain present for an unnatural length of time, (days, weeks, months, or years), this can cause imbalance in the viscus with which that emotion corresponds. Conversely, if a viscus is out of balance for any reason, this can lead to an imbalance in the experiencing of the emotion connected to that viscus. This can become a vicious cycle where the emotion further imbalances an already out of balance viscus, leading to more experience of the emotion, and further imbalance of the viscus. We will discuss this in further detail in the next chapter under irritability and depression.

The Endocrine System & Chinese Medicine

Another notable difference between Chinese and Western physiology is the fact that traditional Chinese medicine does not recognize a separate endocrine system, nor does it describe any endocrine glands. This is not to say that traditional Chinese doctors do not take into account the functions of the endocrine system. They do. Nor is it to say that what Western medicine would call an endocrine dysfunction or imbalance cannot be treated by Chinese medicine. It can. However, the way Chinese medicine describes such hormonal dysfunction is very different. All Western hormonal or endocrine functions are all subsumed under the various functions of the viscera and bowels, channels and network vessels of traditional Chinese physiology. This is just a different map of the same terrain.

One may ask why classical Chinese doctors did not recognize the endocrine system and its complex, hormonal, metabolic control mechanisms. There are, it seems to me, two reasons for this. First, Chinese medical theory is derived from a cosmological, functional theory of how things work in nature which is qualitative, not quantitative. Chinese medicine is based upon the discernment of energetic and functional change, as opposed to chemical and histological change. It is based upon relationships, both within and outside the body, and it tends to look always at the whole picture of the human being within nature, as opposed to any attempt to define smaller and smaller chemical agents (such as hormones) within the body. Western medicine, with its emphasis upon isolation of cellular and molecular structures in the body and specific analysis of chemical components, is opposite in its approach.

Secondly, the Chinese doctor of antiquity had no microscope, at least not until this century, and no lab tests are involved in the traditional Chinese diagnostic process. The Chinese medical system of diagnosis is based upon what is referred to as the four examinations. These include observation with the eyes, auscul-tation/olfaction or listening/ smelling, questioning of the patient in very specific ways, and palpation. This last consists of feeling the pulse at the radial artery, the courses of the channels and network vessels, and/or the abdominal area. From these four examinations, the skilled practitioner of TCM can diagnose the condition of all the viscera and bowels, tissues, and channels of Chinese medicine. What Western science describes as various hormonal or endocrine functions are categorized in Chinese medicine as functions of these tissues, viscera and bowels, or channels. Since hormonal imbalance causes changes which can be noted by these four examinations, the TCM practitioner is able to describe a logical disease mechanism for them within the terminology of Chinese medicine. Such Chinese descriptions do allow for effective treatment without knowledge of the specific chemical substances or hormones involved.

A common problem that the practitioner of Chinese medicine faces with Western clients is the frequent question, "But don't I *really* have a hormone imbalance? Can Chinese medicine treat my hormone imbalance?" This question belies a fundamental belief in the ultimate reality of Western science and the answer to this question is both yes and no. Technically speaking, no, the practitioner of Chinese medicine or TCM is treating a Chinese diagnosis which does not talk about hormones or endocrine glands. However, with correct Chinese medical treatment, a Western diagnosis of a hormone imbalance can be effectively treated. Therefore, the answer is also yes, although, technically and legally speaking, a good practitioner of Chinese medicine cannot say so.

The Mechanism of Menstruation

There are many books available which discuss the hormonal timetable of the menstrual cycle from a Western medical point of view, so that information will not be included here. Chinese medicine has its own theory of the mechanism of menstruation which must be understood if we are also to understand menopause from the Chinese medical perspective.

In Chinese medicine, one name for menstruation is *tian gui*, or heavenly water. Although this term has many interpretations, for the purposes of this discussion of menopause it is identical to menstruation. As stated above, the arrival of *tian gui* is dependent upon a superabundance of blood which brims over every 28 days or so in the healthy adult female.

The creation of blood is the combined work of three viscera, the spleen, heart, and kidneys. The spleen distills the essence of digested food and liquids which it sends to the heart. At the same time, the kidneys provide a small amount of essence which is also sent up to the heart. Remember from the previous sections that

33

essence is the most primal, essential, fundamental of all substances in the body and is, therefore, required as a substrate in all metabolic processes resulting in the creation of a pure substance such as blood. As stated in the Chinese medical classics, the blood is "turned red" in the heart. This means that the final transformation of it occurs in the heart and that the heart then pumps the blood out to nourish the rest of the body.

In order for menstruation to occur, here must be a surplus of blood over and above what is required for survival of the body. Prior to puberty, the organs, in this case especially the spleen and kidneys, are not mature. Consequently the production of qi and blood is also not mature. Therefore, there is not the surplus or excess of blood required for menstruation.

Upon reaching puberty the spleen and kidneys are mature. A superabundance of blood is produced which is stored in the uterus or blood chamber. At this point the uterus is ready for pregnancy. When sufficient blood collects there, and if no pregnancy occurs, this blood brims over, and flows out as menstruation. The menarche, and the onset of every menstrual period thereafter, is called the arrival of *tian gui* or heavenly water.

At this point we must reiterate that up until recent years practitioners of Chinese medicine had no microscopes and no laboratory tests. They did not know about eggs and sperm, estrogen, progesterone, or other hormones. Understanding of the body, while in many ways quite sophisticated, and in all ways quite logical, was based only upon what the doctor could ascertain through the use of the external senses correlated with an understanding of the functions of the viscera and the flow of the energy and blood through the channels and network vessels.

The uterus is given many names in the Chinese literature, among them the fetal palace, the fetal wrapper, the blood chamber, and the wrapper organ. It is a repository—a storage area, and it is considered one of the six extraordinary bowels.[15] The uterus has relationships with a number of viscera and channels which play a part in menstruation and must briefly be described.

The physiological function of the uterus is first dependent upon the kidney and the heart, to which viscera it is connected by two vessels, respectively called the *bao luo* and the *bao mai*.[16] This implies that menstruation is normal when the heart (blood) and kidney (qi and essence) are healthy and in proper communication with the uterus.

Additionally, the spleen plays a role here in that if the spleen is for any reason weak or compromised, there may not be abundant blood created from the digestate and first sent up to the heart to allow for normal menstruation.

Finally, we come to the liver, which plays a major role in the menstrual cycle, having a close relationship with the uterus. In fact, the liver is so important to healthy gynecological function that in some literature it is considered the prenatal viscus in women, as the kidneys are in men. This is because, as stated above, the menstrual blood is the outward physical manifestation of essence in women, and although the uterus is the chamber of blood, it is the liver which stores the blood. That is to say, the

---

[15] Wang, Tao-yang, "A Preliminary Discussion of the Bao Gong, Bao Mai, and Bao Luo", trans. by Zhang Ting-liang and Bob Flaws, *Blue Poppy Essays, 1988*, Blue Poppy Press, Boulder, CO, 1988, p. 17

[16] Ibid., p. 18

liver is responsible for the volume, flow, and regularity of the menstrual cycle and for the blood's nourishing of the sinews and other body tissues as well.

The liver has another function which relates to menstruation as well. It is responsible for the free flow of qi throughout the body and especially in the pelvis. Free flow means regular, smooth, and uninhibited flow. Since the qi commands the blood, these two functions of the liver are closely related. It is said in Chinese: "If the qi moves, the blood moves; if the qi stops, the blood stops." Therefore, if the qi flows unobstructedly, the movement of the blood will also be regular which, in turn, means that menstruation will also be normal, on time, and pain free. And, if the liver stores the blood properly, the menstrual flow will be normal in volume. Anything which disrupts either of these two functions of the liver—storage of the blood and free flow of the qi—is likely to disrupt menstruation and will also have a negative impact upon menopause.

Along with the viscera and bowels, there are several channels which flow through, around, or to the uterus, and may affect its proper functioning. In addition to the *bao luo* and the *bao mai* mentioned above, the kidney, spleen and liver channels all flow through the pelvis with the liver channel directly circulating the genitalia. Even more important are two of the so-called extraordinary vessels which circulate through the pelvis and have an intimate relationship with all female reproductive function. These are the *ren mai*, sometimes called the conception vessel, and the *chong mai*, sometimes called the penetrating vessel. The *ren mai* circulates mostly qi in the area of the anterior midline. Its name, conception vessel, indicates its close relationship to the uterus. The *chong mai* carries mostly blood and circulates in the central core of the body. It is sometimes said that the qi of the *ren mai* commands the blood of the *chong mai* and that together these two vessels are largely responsible for the proper female reproductive function. The *chong mai* can also be called the sea of blood. So one can understand its close connection with the uterus and liver. If any of these channels and vessels are blocked, congested, or deficient, there will be consequences in relationship to menstruation and to menopause.

Now that we have introduced all the players, let us discuss the menstrual cycle itself. A normal menstrual cycle should take 28 days, which is roughly divided into four segments of seven days each. Starting with the onset of the period as day one, during the first week the qi mobilizes the blood in the uterus which is full to overflowing at that point. This blood is moved down and out by the qi. Because the discharge of the blood is the single most important aspect of this segment of the menstrual cycle, the menses are said to correspond to blood.

During the week after menstruation, the blood is relatively empty. It takes blood to enfold and keep the qi down in the body. If the blood is insufficient, the qi, being yang in nature, will rise like a hot air balloon from which the ballast (blood) has been ejected. Therefore, the qi rises toward the upper part of the body. Since blood and essence share a common source and since both are yin substances, because the body's main endeavor at this point is to replace blood and yin, this segment of the menstrual cycle corresponds to yin.

By midcycle or week three, the blood has built back up in volume and is no longer empty. It begins to accumulate in the uterus. The qi has reached its peak in the upper part of the body and begins to be magnetized by the blood in the pelvis back down into the lower half of the body. This downward movement of the qi further mobilizes downward even more blood which accumulates

37

in the uterus. Because yin transforms into yang when it reaches its apogee or extreme, ovulation corresponds to yang.

By week four, the premenstruum, the qi is trying to descend into the lower half of the body in order to move the blood down and out. However, if the women does have not enough blood, what blood there is collecting in the uterus and lower half of the body. This may leave the liver unnourished by sufficient blood. In that case, the liver cannot keep control over the coursing and discharging of the qi. If the liver's coursing and discharging are not normal, then the qi flow is not free. Instead, the qi becomes stagnant and backs up. Most of the symptoms of PMS are related to qi stagnation, accumulation, and counterflow (*i.e.*, erroneous flow). This is why the premenstruum corresponds to qi. For more information on the Chinese conception and treatment of PMS, see Bob Flaws's *Curing PMS Naturally with Chinese Medicine*, also in this series by Blue Poppy Press.

Qi, Blood, Yin & Yang vis-a-vis Menstrual Cycle

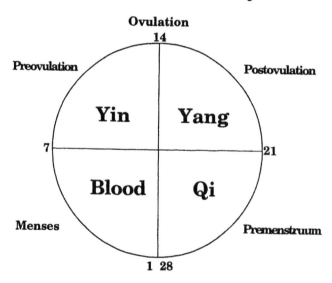

38

Basically, the menstrual cycle is a ceaseless revolution of yin turning into yang and yang turning into yin with the qi rising and falling, moving inward and outward. In Chinese medicine, such transformation and change is controlled by the qi mechanism, and it is the free flow of the qi which keeps the qi mechanism functioning normally. Therefore, qi stagnation is responsible for many menstrual problems, and, as we will see, below, plays a major role in menopausal syndrome, since menopause is simply another of the body's changes and transformations.

Summary

This chapter has introduced many of the basic concepts of Traditional Chinese Medicine: yin/yang theory, the vital substances, the viscera and bowels, channels and network vessels, and the emotions, as well as the Chinese medical view of menstruation. While certainly not an exhaustive explication of Chinese medical theory, the information provided here should allow the reader to enter into the world of Chinese medicine and should make later chapters describing menopausal disorders understandable. If you have trouble understanding information in later these chapters, I suggest that you return to this chapter again for clarification.

MENOPAUSAL SYNDROME:
SIGNS & SYMPTOMS

Menopause is a naturally occurring transition. *As a physiological event, it is not a disease and it need not be accompanied by any discomfort.* Indeed, statistics show that in 20% of all American women, there are no symptoms at all, and in cultures where age brings power and status to women, close to 100% of menopausal women have no reported symptoms.[17]

However, in Western societies where older women are less valued and respected than their younger sisters, approximately 80% of women do have symptoms, ranging from mild and quite transient to severe and debilitating. In Chinese, menopausal symptoms are called *jing duan qian hou zhu zheng* or various diseases arising before or after the cessation of menstruation.

In this chapter we will discuss each of the major symptoms associated with menopause, giving the Chinese medical description of the causation or disease mechanism for each one. Treatments and prevention will be dealt with in later chapters.

The General Picture

In the *Nei Jing (The Inner Classic)*, the first classic of Chinese medicine, it says that at 14 years of age the kidneys are mature,

---

[17] Lyttleton, Jane, *op.cit.*, p. 5

the *ren mai* is free flowing, the *chong mai* is exuberant or full, and the *tian qui* arrives. In other words, a girl reaches puberty and menstruation begins. This is based on a Chinese medical theory which describes the physiological growth, maturation, and decline of reproductive function in women in terms of seven year cycles. Each seven year segment describes a state in the natural history of an individual's kidney function, the foundational viscus of Chinese medical physiology. It is said that at seven times seven years (*i.e.*, at 49 years of age) the kidney qi is debilitated, the *tian gui* is exhausted, and thus the *chong* and *ren* vessels are not nourished, and menstruation ceases.

Since the *tian gui* or menses is the outward manifestation of the essence and of the relationship between the kidney qi and the sea of blood, a weakening of the kidney qi, the essence, and the *chong mai* (sea of blood) will cause the *tian gui* or menstruation to cease. I have mentioned above that the digestive function (read spleen) begins to decline between 35 and 40 years of age. One of the spleen's major functions is to engender the blood and it is mainly blood that makes essence. Therefore, it is this decline in spleen function in the late 30s which directly leads to the debility of the kidneys and insufficiency of essence in the late 40s—not enough blood/essence is produced every 28 days to create an excess which or is discharged as the menses. The menses becomes irregular, the intervals and quantity of blood become erratic, and they eventually stop altogether.

In chapter three on basic Chinese medical theory it was stated that yin and yang must remain in dynamic balance and that blood and qi are a yin/yang pair—the qi moves the blood and the blood is the mother (substrate or root) of the qi. Therefore, as less blood and body fluids (yin) are produced through digestive function, the dynamic balance of qi to blood and yin to yang begins to come out of balance, with qi and yang becoming excess in relationship to blood and yin. This imbalance compounded by each person's constitutional weaknesses is responsible for most of the problems and disease associated with aging. Furthermore, when this process of decline is accompanied by stress, overwork, emotional upsetment, or any organic dysfunction in the body, this disequilibrium between yin and yang is typically worsened.

This disequilibrium often manifests first as kidney yin vacuity.[18] (Vacuity is the technical term when either qi, blood, yin, or yang become empty and insufficient.) However, since yang requires yin as its root, a kidney yin vacuity also eventually leads to a kidney yang vacuity. This is especially so in women in their late 30s and 40s since kidney yang is the prenatal root of the spleen qi and spleen qi begins to weaken in most women by their mid-30s. Thus it is said that spleen qi vacuity may eventually reach kidney yang. Further, since the kidneys are the root of all yin and yang in the body, kidney vacuity, whether yin or yang, may give rise to vacuity and insufficiency in other viscera or bowels. Any viscus may be affected, although different constitutional types tend to manifest the imbalance in different but fairly predictable ways. It is from this general picture that the specific symptoms which we label as part of menopausal syndrome arise. There is, however, one more important concept which we must discuss before we proceed to describe the mechanism for each specific symptom.

Menopause, Stress, and Stagnation

With all the possibilities for problems that the simple facts of aging may lead to, why is it that some women experience few or no symptoms and others suffer severe discomfort? Sometimes the reason is purely genetics. Some of us have a stronger

---

[18] "Yang tends to ever have an excess, yin tends to be ever deficient." This statement is attributed to the great doctor of the Jin/Yuan Dynasty, Xu Dan-xi (1281-1358) and reflects the typical imbalance of yin/yang which he saw in most of his patients. In Chinese medicine it is said that by 40 years of age, yin is half used up.

constitution, better digestion, or stronger kidneys. Another reason is lifestyle, or how well we have taken care of ourselves over the years. Women who take recreational drugs, drink to excess, smoke, eat poorly, and don't exercise can expect a more difficult menopause than their more health conscious sisters. Sociocultural reasons for menopausal syndrome also exist. How the culture in which a woman finds herself views loss of youth and fertility and, more importantly, how a woman views her life purpose in spite of her cultural milieu can greatly affect whether or not she is symptomatic during her menopause.

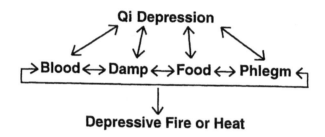

FIGURE 6.
Relationships of the Six Depressions

According to Chinese medicine, unhealthy lifestyle choices as well as sociocultural stressors all contribute to one basic thing that can make the difference between symptoms and no symptoms during menopause, that being stagnation or depression. Stagnation/depression is a concept in Chinese medicine which describes any substance or qi in the body which is not flowing or being transformed properly, and hence getting stuck. Six things can become stagnant or depressed in the body according to TCM: qi, blood, food, dampness, phlegm, or fire. (For a more complete discussion of stagnation/depression in the body, see my previous book, *Better Breast Health Naturally with*

Chinese Medicine, listed in the Suggested Reading section.) Not only will these stagnant or depressed qi and substances cause different types of problems in the body, but they can and usually do interpromote, with one type of stagnation leading to or exacerbating another. (See Figure 6). In the case of menopausal problems, however, the most important of these six is qi. This is so because of all the viscera, qi stagnation most strongly affects the liver and will worsen any problem related to the liver. Since the liver is so strongly connected to the uterus, the *chong* and *ren* vessels, and the menstrual cycle, any liver disharmony caused by qi stagnation will have a strong impact upon menopause. When liver depression/qi stagnation is combined with the normal decline of visceral function associated with the simple fact of being 45 or 50 years old, the process of menopause is not likely to proceed symptom-free. In most American women, liver depression or general qi stagnation symptoms will have been present for some time in the form of digestive difficulties, PMS, breast disease, or frustration and emotional depression before menopause even begins.

The most common reason for liver depression qi stagnation is a disturbance of what are called in Chinese medicine the seven emotions or the seven passions. Another way of stating this is that stress, anger, worry, fear, frustration, boredom, or any other negative emotional state for which a woman has no solution, no outlet, nor the ability to change will cause the qi to stagnate. Since we live in a culture that is mostly unsupportive of older women and where we may find our options growing more limited as we get older, certainly it is no wonder that many women are plagued by such feelings. Add to this the generally high level of stress in our culture for women of all ages, and the prevalence of qi stagnation symptoms this engenders, such as irritability and depression, erratic body pains that come and go, fibrocystic breast disease, chronic digestive disorders, and certain aspects of menopausal syndrome become easy to understand.

45

In the previous chapter I said that the emotions are the subjective mental experience of various manifestations of qi flow as they relate to various organs. What is important about this idea is that *the qi and the mind or emotions are not separate, and what happens to one will happen to the other.* If some aspect of our lives continually makes us feel stuck, dissatisfied, or limited, then over time that is what will happen to our qi as well. This means that our mental/emotional state is most important in either producing or preventing qi stagnation/depression symptoms. We will discuss this point more in the sections on self-help treatment.

Stagnation of qi can cause problems enough by itself—distention and bloating, cramping pain, emotional lability. But as stated above, it will usually complicate other problems that already exist or destabilize any delicate energetic transition that the body is going through, such as menopause. This is because all physiological transitions or transformations, of which menopause is a major example, are dependent upon what is called the qi mechanism. The qi mechanism can only function properly if the qi flows freely. Qi stagnation inhibits this necessary free flow of qi. This fact alone explains why liver depression/qi stagnation complicates any transformation such as menopause and leads to symptoms where they might not otherwise arise.

Warmth is an inherent quality of qi and of life itself, so that if enough of it stagnates in one place for a long enough period of time, it will become hot or transform to (stagnant/depressive) fire. Excessive heat such as this has a number of effects. It dries out the blood and yin of the body which, in menopausal women, are already compromised by the fact of aging. This leads to further imbalance of qi to blood and yin to yang. Further, since blood and yin are required to root or anchor qi and yang, if this imbalance becomes too great, the qi/yang will rise up and to the surface of the body like a hot air balloon. This is how hot flashes, night sweats, headaches, irritability, dry eyes, and certain types of vertigo and insomnia arise.

Another scenario that can happen when depressive/stagnant qi becomes depressive fire is that the blood can become overheated. The qi commands the blood and is responsible for its movement, so that if the qi is hot it may transfer this heat to the blood. Just like water boiling over on the stove, the blood will "boil over" and run recklessly outside its channels. This can cause erratic or excessive bleeding during the period or at unscheduled times between periods. This condition may be further exacerbated by qi vacuity. If there is qi stagnation and blood stasis, fresh qi and blood cannot be created efficiently. Since another inherent function of the qi is to restrain the blood and hold it within its channels, if the qi is insufficient for this job, the blood will not be held in and further bleeding can happen.

In addition to problems with bleeding, long term liver depression/qi stagnation can also become what is called depressive liver fire which can lead to painful breasts, a stuffy, oppressed sensation in the chest, a bitter taste in the mouth, irritability and irascibility alternating with bouts of depression, and possibly bleeding gums, headaches, or toothaches if this fire vents up.

A third possible way in which qi stagnation can aggravate the menopausal situation is if there is already a tendency to kidney yang/spleen yang vacuity. According to the Chinese medical theory of five elements or five phases, liver (wood) must control spleen (earth) (See Figure 7) just as a tree prevents erosion of the soil. If the spleen is already weak, then the liver may overexert this control on the spleen, making it even weaker. The spleen is the organ which, when weak, is responsible for the production of pathogenic phlegm and dampness. If the spleen is made weaker by overcontrol or invasion from a stuck and overheated liver, there will tend to be even more phlegm and dampness, leading to edema, loose stools, obesity, and more seriously, lumps and

47

bumps in the flesh or in the organs. Furthermore, if the liver is overheated, these lumps and bumps can become solidified, like gooey dumplings which harden into bread when steamed or boiled. This is one way that tumors, both benign and malignant, are created. What's worse, if phlegm and dampness are present for any length of time, they will exacerbate qi stagnation, similarly to how a flooded road impedes the normal flow of traffic. Thus, we again see how various stagnant substances or energies, in this case dampness and qi, may interpromote, each making the other worse.

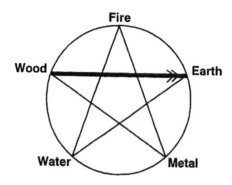

FIGURE 7.
Liver Wood Invades Spleen Earth

Liver depression/qi stagnation will also effect the lungs adversely. According to five phase theory, each viscus is responsible for the control of one other viscus so that none become replete or too strong. (See Figure 8.) It is the lung's job to control the liver. When the liver becomes depressed, this is a species of fullness or repletion. If the liver gets too powerful, it will turn around and attack the lungs which are supposed to keep it in check. (See Figure 9.) In such cases, there may be chronic cough. However, even if there is no cough, weak lungs can contribute to hot flashes and night sweats, the mechanism for which is described in more detail under hot flashes below.

Finally, liver depression qi stagnation can aggravate the heart. Because the relationship of qi and blood is a yin/yang relationship, if the qi (yang) becomes stagnant and hot, the blood (yin) will become evaporated and exhausted. Exhausted blood primarily affects the liver and the heart. The heart is responsible for "treasuring" the spirit (or mind). It is the blood in the heart which is responsible for doing this job. Therefore, if the liver blood and, therefore, heart blood have been exhausted by heat, the spirit will be unable to "rest" or remain calm in the heart. This leads to such symptoms as palpitations, insomnia, restlessness, anxiety, poor memory, emotional lability, and dream-disturbed sleep.

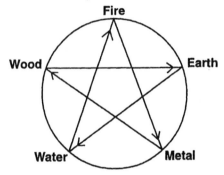

FIGURE 8. Control Cycle of Five Phase Theory

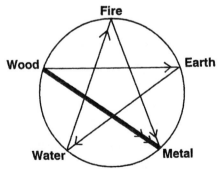

FIGURE 9. Liver Insults the Lung

49

While many of these symptoms may arise without the aggravation of liver depression/qi stagnation, its presence will most assuredly aggravate any tendency that a woman may have toward these symptoms, and its presence or absence will spell the difference between health and the lack of it during menopause. It is rather like the proverbial straw on the camel's back.

The difficulty here is that, according to Chinese medicine, qi stagnation usually worsens with age due to the natural decline of qi, blood, yin, and yang that define aging. All these vital products of physiological activity are necessary for the healthy functioning of the viscera and the free flow of the qi. The good news is that Chinese medicine has techniques for managing and mitigating both the organic as well as the psychological causes of liver depression/qi stagnation.

With all this information about qi stagnation in mind, let us go on to the details of some of the specific symptoms of menopausal syndrome.

Hot Flashes

This is by far the most common symptom women experience during menopause. According to Chinese medicine it is caused by yin vacuity of the kidneys and liver and the consequent rising of liver yang to the upper part of the body. Earlier we spoke of yin being related to water, moistening, coolness, and substance, and yang being related to fire, brightness, and to upward, swift, hot movement. A hot flash is a yang event in the body, the swift upward movement of heat to the surface and especially the chest and head. But this swift erratic movement of heat is due to an underlying emptiness of its opposite, water or yin. Yin is required to enfold, control, root, and lower the yang of the body. If kidney yin is insufficient, yang qi has no root to hold it down, no ballast

50

to keep it from rising, and it therefore floats up out of control to the upper part of the body.

Night Sweats

The mechanism for night sweats is similar to that of hot flashes but with a slight twist. The exterior qi of the body, called *wei* or defensive qi, is the most yang aspect of the qi. It moves quickly, is aggressive, and controls perspiration. During the day it stays on the surface of the body. At night it withdraws into the core of the body to warm and protect the organs. Whether due either to a normal or pathological reason, when this qi moves quickly out to the surface of the body with rising heat, the body fluids in the skin (perspiration) move out with it. Perspiration, according to Chinese medicine, is a pure fluid. It is not a discharge of something foul, fetid, or unnecessary. While normal perspiration with exertion or in hot weather is normal, its excessive, uncontrolled, or untimely loss is not considered healthy. Especially when the body is at rest and not exerting itself, no sweat should appear. Night sweating is a classic symptom of what is called yin vacuity heat or fire. An additional possible mechanism is that when yang qi is weak, which is common in menopausal women, the weakened yang qi cannot do its job of astringing the body surface, which allows body fluids to escape. If both yin and yang are weakened, the situation is therefore that much worse.

Since yin rules or relates to the night hours and the darkness, if the yin is weak, symptoms of its weakness are all the more prevalent during that time. It is during the night especially that yin must do its job of overpowering and enfolding the yang, including the defensive qi. If yin is vacuous and insufficient, it cannot hold and enfold the yang defensive qi which flushes to the surface bringing with it again body fluids in the form of sweat. This is because it is the yang qi which mobilizes and transports fluids. Defensive qi must also keep fluids in the body. If it is weak, the surface is not secured and fluids can escape the surface. When yin and yang are sufficient and in relative balance, night sweating does not occur.

Insomnia

Some women say that the insomnia they have during menopause is due to the night sweats which awaken them, drenched and flushed, having to change their night clothes. Chinese medicine does not necessarily say that it is the night sweats which cause the interruption of sleep so much as that they occur concomitantly.

In the previous chapter we spoke about each of the five major viscera being responsible for, or related to, one of the five spirits or aspects of the psychoemotional make-up. Sleep problems are mostly related to the heart, which "treasures" the spirit and/or the liver which "treasures" the *hun* or so-called ethereal soul. The spirit and the ethereal soul together comprise consciousness. Compared to blood and yin which nourish and root them, they are both yang. If the spirit and ethereal soul cannot be housed properly, sleep will not be calm. The ability of the heart and liver to do this job is directly related to a healthy supply of blood and yin. Systemic blood vacuity due to a decline of spleen and/or kidney function will most often affect the heart or the liver, often resulting in insomnia or dream-disturbed sleep. This again can be seen as the yang counterflowing up due to yin being insufficient to enfold within and hold it down.

Systemic blood vacuity is a common problem in menopausal women. The cessation of the period is, as stated earlier, a sign of the body's declining ability to create blood. It is, therefore, not unreasonable to think that some women might experience symptoms of blood vacuity, insomnia being among them.

Additionally, the blood is a part of the yin of the body and yin is responsible for rest and sleep. If the root of yin, the kidney yin, is vacuous and insufficient, which as we have seen is a common situation in menopausal women, sleep disturbance is a typical consequence of this decline. If there is, as so often happens with American women, the complication of liver depression/qi stagnation, the spleen will also suffer and become weaker, thus reducing blood production to nurture the heart and liver.

To summarize all this, weakening of yin leads to a preponderance of yang and yang is consciousness or wakefulness. Insufficiency of blood prevents the spirit from resting calmly in the heart, and/or the ethereal soul from resting in the liver. This is the basic scenario of insomnia in menopausal women.

Irritability and Depression

These two emotional problems, so common in Western menopausal women, are like two sides of the same coin, and in some women will alternate back and forth, or even occur together. These emotional symptoms are largely due to liver depression/qi stagnation transforming into depressive liver fire over a long period of time.

First the liver qi becomes full or replete, loses its patency and cannot flow freely. If this situation is unresolved, this stuck qi transforms to heat. If this heat remains stuck and congested and is unable to move or change, depression will occur. If the heat comes unstuck and rises in fits and starts, this will often manifest as bursts or fits of anger and irritability which may be inappropriate to the situation. Anger and irritability are hot emotions. These two situations may alternate, or one may be predominant depending upon the case.

Unfortunately, if the liver remains congested and hot, the blood and yin will be further dried out and damaged. This exacerbates the imbalance that already exists creating a vicious cycle. This is one reason that depression is such a difficult symptom to treat effectively. In fact, in cases of severe clinical depression, Western drug therapy is usually necessary while trying to deal with the root of the problem with more natural methods.

Nervousness & Anxiety

Nervousness and anxiety, like insomnia, are related to the heart. As was stated before, the heart must be replete with blood in order for the spirit to rest calmly. When heart blood is vacuous, the spirit has no home or resting place. It therefore flits about like a restless bird, unable to land for long in one place. Our subjective experience of this is a nervous, restless, anxious mental state which may improve or get worse depending upon the level of systemic or heart blood vacuity which is, in turn, related to diet, work, stress, and even how much love is in our life. One highly respected Chinese medical practitioner once told me that one cannot make blood when the heart is longing. Since sufficient blood is such an important factor in women's health this supports the hypothesis that psychoemotional and social factors play an important role in determining a woman's overall health at any time in life.

Fatigue

Fatigue, according to Chinese medicine, is always related to qi vacuity. Movement, activity, and energy to do anything are yang by Chinese definition. Since qi is the aspect of yang which is responsible for motion, action, aliveness, or pep, a shortage of qi will lead to the opposite condition—lethargy, fatigue, and exhaustion. However, once again we must remember the yin/yang relationship of qi to blood. Since blood is the mother of the qi, blood vacuity can also lead to qi vacuity, or exacerbate any tendency to qi vacuity. Therefore, fatigue is also often associated with blood vacuity as well.

The viscera most involved in fatigue are the spleen, lungs, and kidneys. The spleen's job is to transform qi and blood from the essence of digested food and liquids. The lungs' job is to circulate the qi to the body surface and to send it down to the kidneys. The kidneys' job is to grasp or absorb the qi which the lungs descend, energizing the lower body, and to provide the basic fire of life which is the pilot light for the spleen/stomach as well as the libido. The process of creating energy from what we ingest and what we breathe is a process of burning, cooking, or combustion. As has been mentioned several times, the digestive fire of the spleen/stomach begins to weaken at some point in our late 30s or early 40s. Parenthetically, this is why we may put on weight at about that time even though our diet and activity remain the same.

If our diet is not a healthy one or if it requires more fire than what is available in the spleen/stomach, two things can happen. First the kidneys will be required to work harder to provide more heat/qi to assist the spleen/stomach with the logical possibility of them also becoming depleted. If the kidneys cannot make up this deficit or become weak trying to do so, then there will be signs of both spleen qi vacuity and kidney qi vacuity. Since the function that we are talking about here has to do with heat, it will be the yang aspect of the kidneys and spleen that is most likely to be affected. Initially the symptoms may include fatigue, listlessness, fluctuations in appetite, chronic mild diarrhea, or other digestive disturbances. More serious qi vacuity may manifest as anemia, dysfunctional uterine bleeding, prolapse of the stomach, uterus, rectum, or bladder, cold limbs, frequent watery diarrhea, a tendency to easy bruising, nausea, heaviness of the chest or head, or chronic gastroenteritis. These are all spleen qi and yang vacuity signs and symptoms. If the kidneys also become vacuous trying to help out the spleen, further symptoms may include low back pain, sciatica, lack of will power, loss of sex drive, frequent urination, or urinary incontinence. These are typical kidney vacuity signs and symptoms.

Fatigue, therefore, is an initial sign of qi vacuity usually starting with the spleen. This is one reason why a good diet is so important during menopause and all the time really. An entire section will be devoted to diet in Chapter Eight on prevention and self-help.

Palpitations

Palpitations are another heart symptom. However, they can be caused by a number of disease mechanisms. In most menopausal syndrome cases they are due to heart blood vacuity, heart yin vacuity, or heart fire flaring. These may all be aggravated or complicated by flaring upward of liver/stomach heat.

We have discussed heart blood vacuity above in relationship to the spleen. At menopause it is weaker and not supplying the heart with enough raw materials to transform blood properly. Without sufficient blood, the heart qi lacks its foundation causing the function, *i.e.*, the heartbeat, to become irregular. Since qi moves the blood, if heart qi becomes weak, it may not be sufficient to keep the blood flowing and so there are interruptions in the beat.

The source of heart yin vacuity is not related to the spleen but to the kidneys, and to some extent the lungs. In several places above, the kidneys have been mentioned as the source of true yin or original yin. A vacuity of any aspect of kidney energy will almost always affect other organs as well. Also, we have said that the heart and kidney are connected via the internal channels called the *bao luo* and *bao mai* and also via the *chong mai*. Many or even most menopausal symptoms are related, at least in part, to kidney yin vacuity. If the kidney yin is vacuous then the yin of the liver, heart, and lungs also tends to become vacuous. Said more simply, kidney yin vacuity often leads to heart, liver, and lung yin vacuity. In the case of the heart, when kidney yin is vacuous, the kidney and liver yang will rise and overheat the heart. When overheated, the heart qi will move too fast and the heart blood will become dried out from this heat. The exhausted blood will no longer be able to hold onto the qi and perform as its substrate. This coming apart of the qi and blood is experienced as a palpitation. The qi comes apart from the blood which it is moving and skips ahead like a stone skipping over water.

Another possible scenario for menopausal palpitations is heat flushing up from the liver and stomach into the upper body. Heat in the liver is typically due to kidney yin being vacuous and not keeping the liver moist and cool, liver depression qi stagnation transforming to heat, excessive consumption of greasy, spicy foods, or some combination of these factors. Although the stomach can become hot without the liver, the two typically become hot together because of their close relationship. As stated before, when enough heat collects in one place, it rises. If heat from the liver and stomach flush upward, both the heart and lungs can be affected. Another attribute of heat is that it will speed up the movement of qi. In this case the heart qi speeds up and comes apart from the blood which has been dried out or damaged by the heat as well. This can be experienced as a palpitation.

These etiologies for palpitations are related and may combine and interpromote in some women. Again we see the importance of a healthy diet and the control of stress factors which lead to liver depression qi stagnation.

Nausea, Diarrhea & Constipation

These are mostly due to a disharmony between the liver and spleen/stomach. Liver wood must control the unchecked growth of spleen/stomach earth. When the liver becomes depressed and replete, it is common for wood to invade or overcontrol earth. When this happens, the spleen typically becomes vacuous and damp, whereas, the stomach becomes hot and replete along with the liver. Spleen vacuity encumbered dampness leads to loss of appetite, fatigue, and diarrhea. Stomach repletion and upward counterflow causes nausea, belching, and heartburn. Diarrhea can also be aggravated by any tendency to kidney yang vacuity.

The typical cause of menopausal constipation is somewhat different. Earlier it was stated that one of the liver's jobs is to move the qi in a smooth, patent, free-flowing manner. This includes the large intestine qi. When liver qi is congested, it loses its ability to maintain this free flow, often resulting in poor large intestine motility and peristalsis. Add to this a general drying of the yin or moisture in the body and the bowels then are not only difficult to move, but the stools themselves may become dry, hard, and difficult to pass. In TCM terminology, such constipation is described as being due to a combination of liver depression qi stagnation and fluid dryness of the large intestine.

In addition to the qi stagnation and fluid dryness, weakness of kidney yang may also play a role in causing constipation in menopausal and postmenopausal women. The functions of kidney yang include controlling the process that transforms and circulates water through the body. When kidney yang is vacuous, as is common in older people, the process of warming and trans- forming water is weakened. Too much water is excreted by the bladder resulting in clear and copious urination. This disruption in the proper circulation of water in the pelvis dries out the intestines complicating the above mechanism of constipation.

Stiffness & Cramps

According to Chinese medicine, the sinews, i.e., the tendons and ligaments, are nourished by liver blood. When exercising, it is the liver which sends out enough blood to allow the sinews to be strong and flexible. When liver blood becomes vacuous the sinews are not nourished properly, leading to cramping, stiffness, and pain. The mechanism for why liver blood becomes vacuous at menopause has already been discussed in several prior sections above.

Joint Pain

The joints are nourished and kept limber and smooth by the action of the yin fluids of the body. In Chinese medicine, the joints are believed to be ruled by the kidneys and specifically relate to kidney yin. If the true yin or kidney yin becomes vacuous all the yin of the body will be affected, including all body fluids. When these are insufficient, the joints can become painful and lose their flexibility.

In addition, the defensive qi of the body is part of or associated with kidney yang. If kidney yang becomes vacuous and deficient, then it is easier for external evils, such as wind, cold, and dampness, to invade the body and cause impediment and blockage to the channel qi. Thus limb and joint pain occurring around menopause may be due to either yin or yang vacuity, and, in fact, is often due to a combination of both. (Pain in the spinal vertebrae due to bone demineralization is covered below.)

Vaginal Dryness

The vagina is also kept moist, soft, and lubricated by the body fluids. Additionally, the genitals are ruled by the kidney and liver. If kidney/liver yin is vacuous and insufficient, the body fluids in the genital area will be affected. If there is also liver qi stagnation, the genitals will tend to become dried out due to transformative heat in the liver channel, which directly circulates the genitalia. This not only causes dryness but chronic inflammation and/or itching. Persistent vaginal discomfort may also contribute to loss of interest in sex.

Osteoporosis

According to TCM, the kidneys rule the bones, teeth, head hair, ears, and the marrow of the spinal cord and brain. If symptoms arise in these areas of the body, the Chinese medical practitioner always investigates for kidney involvement. Since we know the kidneys are already in a natural state of decline by the time of menopause, the bones will also be declining. In Chinese medicine, it is said that the essence is stored in the marrow and that the marrow becomes the bones. Essence is yin when compared to qi. But essence is actually made out of both yin and yang. Around menopause, typically both liver blood and kidney yang are vacuous and insufficient, and it is this liver blood, kidney yang vacuity which is primarily responsible for postmenopausal osteoporosis. Fortunately, there are many things a woman can do to prevent bone demineralization and avoid osteoporosis. These are discussed in the chapters on prevention (8) and osteoporosis (12).

Abnormal or Excessive Bleeding

Chinese medical theory describes abnormal bleeding of any type as due to one or a combination of three causes: heat, blood stasis, or qi vacuity. In menopausal women, abnormal uterine bleeding is typically due to some combination of at least two of these, and in some cases all three. As described earlier on page 48-49, long term qi stagnation may lead to what is called depressive heat causing the blood to boil over and run recklessly outside its pathways. Additionally, heat due to yin emptiness, which is so common in menopausal women, may worsen any tendency to depressive heat. Secondly, since it is qi which holds the blood within its pathways, vacuous qi may be too weak to perform this function, allowing the blood to fall or leak out. Finally, blood stasis creates blockage causing the blood to flow outside its normal pathways rather like a traffic jam with cars driving down the shoulders or median strip in order to keep moving.

Loss of Sex Drive

This is a very upsetting symptom for most women and may adversely affect relationships with husbands or lovers. Vaginal discomfort and dryness may play a role here, but other disease mechanisms also usually play a part. Sexual desire is a function of kidney yang—the fire of the kidneys, sometimes called the *ming men huo*, or life gate fire. Due to spleen qi vacuity beginning in the mid-thirties eventually reaching kidney yang, many menopausal women suffer from at least some kidney yang vacuity. Therefore, a woman feels no desire for sex. Happily once again, such perimenopausal kidney yang vacuity with attendant loss of sex drive can be both prevented and treated with Chinese medicine.

Early Menopause & Artificial Menopause

Although not specifically symptoms of menopause, early menopause and artificial menopause are not uncommon phenomenon in our culture and deserve some discussion. Early menopause is described by Western medicine as menopause which occurs prior to the age of 40, having many potential causes. Having made a diagnosis of early menopause, Western medical practitioners usually prescribe estrogen replacement therapy for such women. According to Chinese medical theory, early menopause indicates that a woman has aged prematurely. That is to say, her biological age has exceeded her chronological age. Usually this indicates decline in kidney essence or both kidney yin and yang. If the woman has not gone completely through menopause but is still menstruating at least sporadically, Chinese medicine can often regulate menstruation. Although many women may not particularly care to have their regular monthly periods, menopause does signal the end of fertility and the possibility of bearing children. Therefore, most women concerned about early or premature menopause are really concerned about infertility. When Chinese medical treatment is effective in restoring regular menstruation, it means that Chinese medicine has succeeded in rolling back the biological age of these women resulting in their being biologically younger.

Surgical menopause is menopause due to the removal of the uterus and, in some cases, the ovaries as well. Obviously Chinese medicine cannot reverse surgical menopause. However, because the monthly discharge of blood is one way the body rids itself of static blood, also read dry blood, dead blood, and malign blood, surgical menopause may result in the accumulation of static blood in the lower abdomen, and this may lead, in turn, to the formation of abdominal masses or neoplasms. Appropriate Chinese medical treatment can at least mitigate the effects of such blood stasis and its potential consequences in women who have undergone surgical menopause.

Radiation and chemotherapy can also cause artificial menopause because they injure and deplete the essence and blood. Frequently this is accompanied by various menopausal complaints. Chinese medicine sees both these Western therapies as being very hot, and their side effect is to often cause heat in the blood. Chinese medical treatment can help replenish the essence and blood damaged by these therapies and clear heat from the blood, thus controlling any negative side effects from these therapies.

Other Symptoms

Other symptoms that occasionally appear with menopause may include dizziness, vertigo, headaches, blurring vision, tinnitus, excessive thirst, edema, cold limbs, low back pain, weight gain, poor appetite, and memory loss. These are all related to one or more of the basic diagnostic patterns of disharmony which account, alone or in combination, for menopausal discomfort. These patterns are discriminated in detail in the next chapter.

THE TCM DIAGNOSIS OF MENOPAUSAL
SYNDROME PATTERNS OF DISHARMONY

Diagnosis in TCM is based on the discrimination of profession-ally recognized, named patterns of disharmony. Traditional Chinese diagnostic patterns are differentiated based on signs and symptoms, observation of the tongue, and palpation of the pulse, abdomen, channels and vessels. They are not based on laboratory tests. Traditional Chinese patterns of disharmony are usually directly descriptive of the patient's experience of their disease.

Also, the descriptive patterns used in Chinese medicine are derived from a direct observation of phenomena in the natural world. Let us take for example the pattern called "wind." As a natural phenomenon, wind comes out of nowhere, is fast moving, comes and goes in fits and starts, and causes things to move, shake, tremble, or change shape. Wind as a diagnostic pattern describes exactly the same qualities. Wind diseases come on rapidly, move quickly, possibly from one part of the body to another, can come and go unexpectedly, and cause involuntary movement. Further, because wind manifests in heaven or the sky, wind diseases also typically manifest in the upper part of the body.

TCM diagnostic patterns are classified in several ways. The first way patterns may be subdivided is whether they are viscera and bowel patterns, channel and network vessel patterns, or patterns related to specific tissues in the body. The second subdivision is slightly more complex, dividing patterns by what are called the eight principle: hot and cold, vacuity and repletion, external and internal, yin and yang. Thirdly, patterns are subdivided according to whether they involve the body humors: qi, blood, body fluids, and essence. Finally, patterns may be classified according to five phase or five element theory.

In actual practice, these pattern categories are combined when diagnosing a single patient thus giving a great deal of texture and complexity to pattern identification. Each individual pattern has its professionally agreed upon signs and symptoms. However, real life patients almost always suffer from a combination of two or more such patterns of disharmony and so their signs and symptoms are likewise a mixture. Textbooks must describe these patterns as distinct, but few patients present such neatly packaged signs and symptoms. For this reason, TCM practitioners practice for years before really developing the skill to move from such simple textbook discriminations to diagnosing complex real life patients.

Happily, in menopausal syndrome only a few of these patterns predominate. That is because disharmony in women's bodies tend to arise in specific ways at specific times in our lives depending upon our constitutional make-up. In fact, based upon a woman's constitution at 30 or 35, a good practitioner of Chinese medicine should be able to predict quite accurately what type of menopausal problems, if any, a woman is likely to experience and perhaps offer her preventive suggestions.

Below are the major patterns of disharmony which account for most menopausal symptoms, with a description of the signs and symptoms defining each pattern. However, remember that, as just stated, these patterns can, and often do combine with each other or with other patterns related to a woman's constitutional tendencies to make the overall picture of a woman's health more

66

complicated. Rarely will a woman's situation be as simple as one or another of these patterns alone.

Liver Blood, Kidney Yin Vacuity

Liver blood, kidney yin vacuity is the main direct mechanism for the cessation of menstruation. Menses stop because there is insufficient liver blood and kidney yin or essence to support it. In women where this dual vacuity is more severe, however, it may also result in other signs and symptoms. These include:

-hot flashes/sweating, especially in the upper body
-headaches, blurred vision, dizziness, vertigo, tinnitus,
    spots in front of the eyes
-weakness/soreness of lower back or legs
-constipation
-thirst or dry mouth
-insomnia or dream-disturbed sleep

Tongue: red, with little or no coating or a dry scant yellow
    coating
Pulse: fine, bowstring, and rapid

These signs and symptoms are due to a drying up of yin below. This causes fluid dryness constipation and weakness or soreness of the low back and legs due to lack of blood nourishing the sinews. This also results in yang floating upward due to its lack of root in the yin below. This results in hot flashes, night sweats, dizziness, blurred vision, insomnia, and a dry mouth. This is one of the most common menopausal patterns of disharmony. It arises due to the spleen no longer creating a superabundance of blood and blood and yin being used up by the act of living. Typically, no matter what other patterns may complicate an individual woman's menopause syndrome, the vast majority of women with menopausal complaints exhibit this pattern as well.

67

Ascendant Liver Yang Hyperactivity

Ascendant liver yang hyperactivity is derived from liver depression qi stagnation which undergoes transformation due to the previous pattern. The pure signs and symptoms of this pattern are:

-dizziness and vertigo
-tinnitus and red eyes
-menopausal migraines
-a bitter taste in the mouth
-irritability and even irascibility
-hot flashes and sweats
-profuse menstrual flow due to heat in the blood
-lingering menstrual flow or spotting

Tongue: red
Pulse: bowstring and rapid

These signs and symptoms describe more forceful ascension of yang to the upper part of the body than the previous pattern. The previous pattern's signs and symptoms describe empty heat rising whereas ascendant liver yang hyperactivity symptoms are due to yang repletion and counterflow. The mechanism for the signs and symptoms are not different as both have to do with a flushing up of yang. The difference lies in degree. This technical difference is important when it comes to TCM therapeutics. Often kidney yin, liver blood vacuity is complicated by ascendant liver yang hyperactivity.

Spleen & Kidney Yang Vacuity

In this pattern, symptoms mostly reflect cold and dampness accumulating in the body due to an inability of spleen and kidney yang to transport and transform body fluids. The signs and symptoms are:

-pale complexion
-limbs and body cold and an aversion to cold
-lower back painful and/or cold
-loss of appetite
-clear copious urine or
-very scant urine accompanied by edema
-abdominal distention
-early morning diarrhea or tendency to loose stools
-loss of sex drive
-obesity

Tongue: pale, swollen with a white or wet coating
Pulse: deep, weak, and/or slow

In actual clinical fact, fatigue is the main symptom of spleen vacuity, while low back pain, cold feet, nocturia, and decreased libido are the main symptoms of kidney yang vacuity in perimenopausal women.

Accumulation of Phlegm & Stagnation of Qi

This pattern is due to the decline of spleen function in its processing of liquids. As mentioned above, liver depression qi stagnation typically leads to spleen vacuity and dampness. Likewise, decline of kidney yang also leads to spleen vacuity since the root of the spleen's ability to transform and transport is derived from the heat of the kidneys. It is said in Chinese medicine that the spleen is the root of phlegm production. Phlegm is due to the congelation of dampness. This is aggravated by any tendency towards liver heat which brews the fluids cooking them into phlegm. Once phlegm is created it tends to block the flow of qi, thus aggravating liver qi. It may also obstruct what in Chinese medicine are called the orifices of the heart. This results in various mental/emotional symptoms. Although this pattern rarely causes menopausal signs and

69

symptoms by itself, it does often complicate and aggravate all the other, more common patterns associated with menopausal complaints. The signs and symptoms of accumulation of phlegm and stagnation of qi are:

- -stuffy chest or "chest oppression"
- -depression
- -fear and anxiety
- -palpitations
- -insomnia
- -copious mucous
- -a possible lump in the throat
- -nausea or vomiting
- -obesity

Tongue: darkish with a turbid, greasy coating
Pulse: slippery and bowstring

Heart Blood, Spleen Qi Vacuity

Spleen qi catalyzes the creation of heart blood. If the spleen qi is vacuous, over time heart blood will also become vacuous and insufficient. Constant worry and too much thinking may also lead to this condition. The symptoms of heart blood, spleen qi vacuity are:

- -palpitations and shortness of breath
- -anxiety or emotional instability
- -loss of memory
- -insomnia and/or excessive dreams
- -pale or yellowish complexion
- -tendency to fatigue
- -itchy skin

Tongue: pale and flabby with teeth indentations on the sides
Pulse: fine and weak or vacuous

Heart Yin & Blood Vacuity

This pattern is due to the heart yin and blood not being transformed and thus failing to nourish and quiet the heart spirit. Because heart yin is rooted in kidney yin, decline of liver and kidney yin may result in heart yin vacuity. And because the spleen and liver are the two viscera which participate in the control of blood, if spleen qi no longer engenders the blood and the liver no longer stores blood as efficiently as previously, heart blood may become vacuous. In addition, since heart blood and yin are both species of yin they are mutually interdependent.

The signs and symptoms of heart yin and blood vacuity primarily have to do with the blood and yin's failure in nourishing the function of the heart and the heart spirit. This results in:

-dream-disturbed sleep
-palpitations
-loss of memory
-insomnia

If heart yin vacuity predominates, the signs and symptoms will be:

-restlessness
-heat in the palms, soles, and center of the chest
-afternoon low-grade fever
-night sweats
-racing of the heart

Tongue: If heart blood vacuity predominates, the tongue is pale. If heart yin vacuity predominates, the tongue is red.
Pulse: If heart blood vacuity predominates, the pulse is fine and forceless. If heart yin vacuity predominates, the pulse is fine and rapid.

71

Heart & Kidneys Not Interacting

This pattern describes a situation where, due to loss of inter-promotion and mutual restraint of fire and water in the body, a woman experiences hot symptoms in the upper body and cold symptoms in the lower. Fire blazes up and water dribbles down. According to five phase theory, the water of the kidneys should maintain communication with and control over the fire in the heart. When this communication is lost, the following symptoms will appear:

-insomnia
-nervousness and anxiety
-palpitations
-frequent dreams
-leukorrhea or excessive vaginal discharge
-incontinence or dribbling urination
-uterine bleeding

Tongue: red tip, apically fluted, scant coating
Pulse: fast, floating, or surging

The difference between this heat above and cold below and that of the previously described patterns is that the signs and symptoms of heat primarily manifest as disruptions in heart function according to TCM. This pattern therefore, specifically describes a heart/kidney imbalance as opposed to a more general yin/yang disequilibrium.

This pattern differs from the preceding patterns in that there is vacuity fire flaring upward in the heart disturbing the spirit. Whereas in the preceding pattern, the spirit is simply mal-nourished.

Kidney Yin & Yang Vacuity

This pattern is again a mixture of both hot and cold symptoms. It often appears as hot symptoms above and cold symptoms below. Since the yin of the kidneys is weak, whatever weak yang there is in the body is not rooted and floats up, leaving the lower body yang vacuous and, therefore, cold. Compared to the previous pattern, the symptoms of spirit unrest are less severe and the symptoms of cold and kidney vacuity below are more severe. Varying symptoms may arise including:

-cold lower limbs; low back feels cold
-body feels like it is sitting in cold water from the
    waist down
-afternoon flushes of the face, neck, ears
-dry eyes and throat
-headaches, vertigo
-aversion to cold
-sweating palms, face, or chest
-abnormal uterine bleeding
-polyuria and nocturia
-low back weakness and weak knees
-loss of sex drive
-fatigue

Tongue: usually pale, possibly with a wet coating
Pulse: Here the pulse could be deep and weak or fine and fast depending upon whether yin or yang is more compromised.

Chinese Patterns & Western Women

Modern TCM gynecology texts differentiate menopausal syndrome into the several patterns listed above. However, as previously mentioned, one rarely sees such discrete patterns in individual patients and especially not in Western women. Rather, most menopausal Western women tend to have some element of liver

73

blood, kidney yin *and* yang, heart blood, and spleen qi vacuity with floating yang in the upper body and fluid dryness in the lower, all further complicated by liver depression qi stagnation. Symptoms of all these patterns appear in different combinations depending upon a specific woman's constitution, current stress level, diet, and many other factors. The most common symptoms of this composite pattern are:

-hot flashes and night sweats
-palpitations
-low back pain, possible sciatica
-irritability and emotional instability
-fatigue
-constipation, or alternating constipation and diarrhea
-insomnia
-bleeding gums
-dysfunctional uterine bleeding
-polyuria, nocturia
-loss of sex drive

Tongue and pulse: Because this combination pattern can arise with so many variations it is impossible to suggest only one tongue or pulse conformation.

Once women go through menopause, their consumption of yin slows down drastically. No longer losing blood on a monthly basis they cannot really afford to lose, they retrench and consolidate their yin. If menopause proceeds smoothly and is not allowed to drag itself out, most women have few menopausal complaints and can live another twenty years or more before beginning again to feel marked symptoms of decline. There are many preventive therapies and lifestyle modifications that can help menopause to proceed more quickly and smoothly. Additionally, Chinese medicine offers a number of therapeutic options for women who need professional support during this time. The following chapters describe these preventive and remedial options.

74

HEALTHY MENOPAUSE: A SECOND SPRING

Going through menopause does not automatically mean that symptoms will arise. Just on the physical level, if a woman's diet is good, if she exercises moderately but regularly, if she limits stress in her life where possible and has an effective way of dealing with stress when it does arise, that woman is less likely to experience symptoms when she reaches menopause or at any other time for that matter! There are women who sail through menopause with little or no discomfort whatsoever.

It is important to reiterate that menopause is not a disease. Quite the contrary, it is an intelligent homeostatic mechanism on the part of a woman's body. We have discussed this in earlier chapters but this is such an important and, for Western women, such a novel statement, that it bears review.

As was previously stated, after the age of 35 or so the digestion naturally begins to lose its efficiency. This means the spleen/stomach is less able to create qi and blood from the refined essence of the food and liquids. Because there is no longer a surplus of qi and blood being transformed by the spleen/stomach, as time goes by there is less and less postnatal or acquired essence to be sent to the kidneys for storage. Again, this is like capital and interest. If the body is not creating postnatal essence (interest), it will have to begin dipping into its finite supply of prenatal essence (capital). This at least partially describes the aging process, but need not necessarily imply disease symptoms.

75

The kidneys as well as the spleen/stomach begin to decline in function in our late 30s. This will also have a negative impact on the creation of blood since the kidneys along with the spleen and heart participate in its production. It is said that the blood and essence share a common source—the kidneys. This implies that each month when a woman menstruates, some essence is lost with her menstrual blood. Indeed, the menstruate is the outward physical manifestation of essence in a woman. Once her body is no longer producing a surplus of blood and essence, this situation of monthly loss cannot go on indefinitely if she is to remain healthy. After a certain age menstruation is draining her kidneys and exhausting the *chong* and *ren* vessels.

At some point, the body recognizes what is going on and, to slow down the loss of essence and blood, shuts down the monthly menstrual cycle. This homeostatic mechanism is the menopause. It is a healthy and positive response of the body to the natural aging process and allows a woman the possibility of remaining in relatively good health with very slow decline for another 20 to 30 years. If there were no menopause, a woman would age much more quickly due to the continual drain of blood and essence which are the nutritive (yin) foundation of the body.

Let's now move on to what things a woman can do for herself to facilitate the process of menopause and ensure that it proceeds smoothly and without discomfort.

8

PREVENTION & SELF-HELP

Menopausal women need not believe that they are doomed to years of hormonal nightmare. Premenopausal women need not anticipate with dread the menopausal years. All women, however, need to act with intelligence to bring their being into a state of health whereby menopausal discomforts may be reduced or eliminated. On the one hand, it is important for all of us to recognize and accept the facts of aging and decline. These are part of the human condition and used to be accepted as such. On the other hand, we need not believe that either menopause or the postmenopausal years doom us to several decades of excessive and continual suffering. It is up to us to determine how these years will be experienced, and it is up to us to act upon that determination. The rest of this book gives suggestions for perimenopausal women (the years on either side of menopause) to improve their bodies' overall health, increase their production of qi and blood, and reduce stress and therefore liver depression qi stagnation, thereby improving their chances for a healthy and symptom free menopause and slower decline in the post-menopausal years.

Since aging according to Chinese medicine has much to do with the state of the kidneys and since so many signs and symptoms of menopausal syndrome are directly related to decline of the kidneys, most of the suggestions classically given to perimenopausal women have to do with maintaining the health of the kidneys. In this book, however, equal attention will be given to the health of the liver, which, in my opinion, is equally important in our culture and at this time in history.

The order in which these suggestions are given does not imply an order of importance. All of them are important, but few of us have the time to do everything that is described here as useful. As you read, note which suggestions you personally resonate with and can accept or incorporate into your life and which you cannot, and why. Consider that perhaps the ones you have the most resistance to may be the most important for you.

Remember that these suggestions are given with the under-standing that not all of them will be or even should be taken. Few of us are capable of doing everything that we know is good for us, and moderation even in the things that are good for us is probably a sign of a relaxed and basically healthy attitude to life. Try to develop habits or choose regimes that fit into your life without creating more stress. If you find that you feel you cannot make any of these options a part of your life, you may want to think about whether your lifestyle is a fundamentally healthy one and if some basic changes need to be made.

Exercise

Everyone needs exercise to maintain health. Exercise is important for stress reduction, weight control, and cardiovascular health. To be effective for cardiovascular health, exercise need not be overly strenuous. Studies done recently have shown that moderate exercise may be just as beneficial to the heart and lungs as vigorous exercise.[20] Also, research just publicized this month has indicated that women who exercise regularly have

---

[20] Anon, "Build Exercise into Your Lifestyle", *Staying Well Newsletter*, American Chiropractic Assoc., May-June 1989, p. 1

lower rates of breast and possibly other cancers.[21] It is also true that for weight reduction, more calories are burned with more vigorous exercise or a combination of moderate and vigorous exercise during the same session. But whether you are a vigorous or moderate exerciser, it is, as the advertisement goes, very important to "just do it" and on a regular basis.

If you are not interested in sports, or in joining an aerobics class, many normal daily activities can be exercise. Housework, yard work, walking to work or to the bus stop, washing the car, all these are exercise. If you are really motivated, walking or biking to work has the added benefit of helping the environment and saving money on gasoline, parking, and auto maintenance. If none of these activities are possible on a regular basis, try finding a walking, jogging, or bicycling buddy. This will give you the incentive to keep up your schedule since there is another person depending on you for your support. This also helps prevent boredom since it gives you someone to talk to while you're exercising. However a woman goes about getting sufficient regular exercise, a number of benefits will accrue to her, all of which are valuable.

For menopausal women, regular exercise is even more important because lowered levels of blood estrogen are related to an increased risk for cardiovascular disease in women over 50 years of age. *Exercise has been shown to be of benefit in reducing cardiovascular disease.*

Another continuing issue for many women after menopause which is related to exercise is weight control. Some Western

---

21   "Warding Off Breast Cancer", *Newsweek*, Vol.134, #14, p. 58.

doctors believe that this struggle with weight is related to the fact that the estrogen which our body continues to produce after menopause requires fat cells for its metabolism and use by the body. This increase in fat cells is the body's way of trying to create more estrogen as blood levels of estrogen begin to drop.[22] *Exercise has always been an important part of weight control programs, and can help the menopausal woman control this tendency to store excessive fat.*

By this I do not mean that women can or even should try to regain or maintain the figure of a sixteen year old. This is neither a possible nor a healthy endeavor. It may even be true that a body with a *little* extra fat on it is healthier than a very thin one. Remember that from a Chinese medical point of view, substance is yin, and yin is what most menopausal women are lacking. Excessive or neurotic thinness can exacerbate yin vacuity. Too much substance becomes pathogenic dampness and is also not healthy, but as a culture we often err to the side of trying to be too thin for our own health.

The third reason why exercise is important is that it helps control stress and minimizes stagnation. Stagnation is the opposite of movement, so the external movement provided by exercise circulates the qi and blood and any other substance in the body tissues which may be stuck. If the qi is flowing freely, the emotions are more likely to be balanced and flowing freely as well. If the emotions are flowing freely, there is less tendency for the qi to stagnate in the first place. Women with a tendency to irritability, anger, or moodiness will benefit greatly from regular exercise and so will those around them!

Also, from the point of view of Chinese medicine, regular exercise stimulates the spleen and strengthens the lungs. Since we know

---

[22]   Greenwood, Sadja, op.cit. p. 21

that the spleen is less active as we grow older, anything which helps the spleen function will improve digestion, help transform dampness and phlegm, and boost the general energy level. Strengthening the lungs is also important because, according to five phase energetics, it is the lungs which must keep the liver in check. This prevents liver qi from becoming full, rising up out of control, or venting itself on other viscera, most commonly the spleen and stomach.

As mentioned above, *recent studies reported in the media show that women who exercise regularly lower their chance of developing breast cancer.* The more years of exercise, the more this protection increases.[23] This makes perfect sense from the information in the above paragraph and in the previous chapter on Chinese medical theory. If the spleen is strengthened by regular exercise, there is less likelihood of the production of phlegm and dampness which can congeal into neoplasms. Also, exercise helps prevent blood stasis which is, according to Chinese medical theory, a contributing factor in many types of cancer. Considering this, exercise contributes to longevity by helping prevent cancer as well as a healthier menopause.

Finally, many studies have been done which show that *weight bearing exercise, even of a relatively moderate type, such as walking, swimming, or dancing, will increase bone calcium levels of postmenopausal women, and help prevent bone demin-eralization or osteoporosis.* Since 90% of all cases of osteoporosis in the U.S. occur in postmenopausal women,[24] it is easy to see why exercise is so important. Risk factors for osteoporosis include:

---

[23]   *Op. cit.*, p. 58.

[24]   Gambrell Jr., Don R., *op.cit.*, p. 22

-Caucasian or Asian heritage
-a family history of osteoporosis
-lifelong low calcium intake
-early menopause
-surgical removal of ovaries at a young age
-a sedentary lifestyle
-no children
-excessive alcohol, salt, or caffeine intake
-cigarette smoking
-excessive protein intake
-treatment with steroid drugs
-hyperthyroidism

Obviously, the more of these risk factors anyone has in their lifestyle or medical history, the higher is their risk for osteoporosis and, concurrently, the more is their need for regular weight bearing exercise. Other preventive therapy to lower the risk of osteoporosis will be discussed in the section on orthomolecular or micronutrient therapy and in Appendix II.

For some of us, exercise comes naturally and is not a difficult part of our lives. Unfortunately, it is often the people who resist exercise that need it the most. For example, people with an overabundance of pathological dampness and phlegm in the form of overweight find it difficult to exercise energetically. Yet, because exercise mobilizes and melts dampness and phlegm, it is a very important part of therapy for anyone with this type of problem. Since the sedentary lifestyle that many women have by this time in life may lead to overweight, regular exercise becomes all the more important. If you are a person for whom the commitment to exercise is difficult to make, try taking it in smaller, simpler steps. Don't create an exercise program that is unrealistic. You will not stick to it and this will just convince you all the more that you cannot do it. Try parking your car closer to home and farther from work or try taking the bus and walking to and from the bus stop. Find a local class in something you've always wanted to learn like tennis, ice skating, or belly dancing. There are also many types of exercise tapes available if you prefer to exercise alone and in the privacy of your home. These can usually be rented from libraries and video rental stores so that you can get an idea of what sort of tapes you like before making any financial commitment. The possibilities for exercise are really limitless. The important thing is that you find something that you like and can stick to on a regular basis.

Stretching

Although stretching is really a type of exercise, I have given it its own section because it is important for different reasons than those listed above and because I wish to emphasize its importance. The practice of stretching can be included either as part of an overall exercise program or as a separate regimen, but it should not be overlooked in any case. In fact, it is my belief that if you cannot discipline yourself to any other type of exercise, stretching may be the most important type of exercise to get.

The reason that I say this is that as we age our bodies become less flexible. This is due to the natural decline of yin associated with aging. Yin is the fluid and blood that keep the tendons, ligaments, bones, and joints supple and flexible. As yin is lost, there is the natural tendency for these tissues to become dry and stiff. If these tissues are stretched and kept as supple as possible on a daily basis, they will be more likely to remain that way for a longer time.

Additionally, because of this decline of yin and consequent stiffness, joint and muscle aches and pains are common complaints of older people. Gentle, regular stretching can be a great help in preventing the debilitating effects and financial drain of chronic pain syndromes related to aging.

There are many ways to go about stretching. Most city recreation departments have yoga classes. There are a number of good yoga books and video tapes as well, although if you wish to take up yoga regularly, I suggest taking at least a few classes initially so that you do not injure yourself by wrong postures or over-stretching. There are also books available on just plain stretching which are quite good. I have listed several books in the Suggested Reading section which may be of help.

If you are going to aerobics or dance classes, or using exercise videos as your main form of exercise, be sure that there is at least a minimal stretching component to them. One of the healthiest postmenopausal women I know, despite a double mastectomy eight years ago, is a dance teacher who stretches and exercises daily. She is a reminder to me not to underrate the importance of exercise for overall health.

Finally, whatever type of exercise you choose to do, there are a few things to remember:

- Regularity or consistence is more important than vigorousness.
- It is important to pick something that you enjoy doing.
- Regular stretching should be a part of every exercise regime.
- The quality and comfort of your golden years will be directly related to the health of your body, which will be greatly improved by regular exercise.

Abdominal Self-Massage

Self-massage may sound strange to some women, but its efficacy for improving health has been known in Japan for centuries. Although there are self-massage regimes for the entire body, the abdomen or *hara* is considered especially important. In Japanese,

84

the *hara* is the entire soft portion of the belly. It stretches from just below the diaphragm to the top of the pubic bone. In Asia this area is considered a person's vital center. Anatomically, it contains all the vital organs of Oriental medicine except the heart and lungs. In traditional Japanese medicine, it is believed that a healthy *hara* is the sign of and key to health in general.

Traditionally, the *hara*'s health is ascertained through palpation (touch). Pain, lumps and bumps, abnormal muscular tension, abnormal pulsation, and hyper- or hypotonicity may all be signs that the internal organs are imbalanced or dis-eased. A corollary of this is that, if pain or other abnormal findings in the abdomen are relieved, imbalance or disease of the internal organs these signify will simultaneously be relieved.

Happily, one can not only diagnose the balance and imbalance of the viscera and bowels by palpating the abdomen but one can directly treat these viscera and bowels with nothing more than pressure applied with one's own hands. Many famous Japanese therapists, such as Kiyoshi Kato and Naoichi Kuzome, treat the full range of human disease primarily through *hara shiatsu* or abdominal massage.

The stomach, spleen, and intestines are of primary importance to health according to Traditional Chinese Medicine. If the stomach and intestines are functioning normally, abundant qi and blood will be produced. Likewise, the clear yang (consciousness and abundant energy) will be upborne and the turbid yin (waste products) will be downborne for excretion and evacuation. This upbearing of the clear and downbearing of the turbid is called the qi mechanism. A healthy qi mechanism insures that the qi and blood will travel unobstructedly in their proper directions and to their proper destinations, thus nourishing and empowering all the functions and tissues of the organism. When the qi mechanism and the stomach and intestines are functioning in a healthy way, neither qi, blood, dampness, phlegm, food, or fire will have an opportunity to become stagnant and thus give rise to disease. Further, a healthy qi mechanism insures that the change and transformation of menopause can take place without hitch or hang-up.

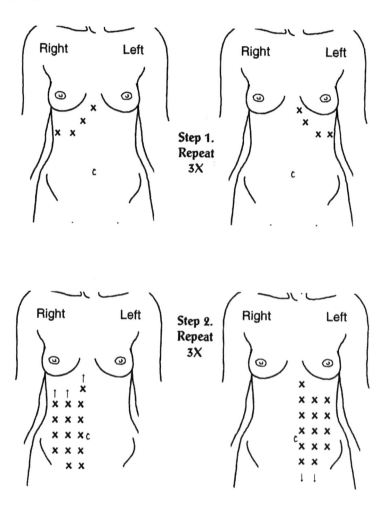

Step 1.
Repeat
3X

Step 2.
Repeat
3X

The intestines or bowels only function normally when they are free flowing according to traditional Chinese medical theory. This means that the bowels function correctly when they constantly send down the turbid, the residue, for excretion. When this residue or turbidity is retained within the organism, it gives rise to numerous disease mechanisms. It is the qi which empowers peristalsis and moves the turbid down through the intestines.

Abdominal self-massage is one easy but nonetheless effective way to keep the qi and blood in the internal organs flowing unobstructedly and the bowels from becoming stagnant with retained turbidity. Although *hara shiatsu* is often performed professionally in Japan by trained therapists, it is easy to do a simpler version oneself and is all the more effective when done on a daily basis.

One begins by lying on their back with their knees drawn up. If the feet are spread slightly apart, the knees can fall together in the center and hold themselves up without any further effort. Next one presses with the flats of the fingers of both hands under the right ribs. One begins pressing as one exhales. Continue to press and exhale to a count of six. When inhaling, move the fingers down and over to the sides of the rib cage and exhale and press again. Do this three times until one winds up pressing under the floating ribs at their sides. See the previous page for a visual image.

Next go back to the midline beneath the ribs and repeat this sequence moving to the left in three exhalations. During this first pass over the hypochondrium, the pressure should not be too strong. Now repeat this entire sequence two more times, each time pressing a little harder.

At first, it is not uncommon to experience pain, resistance, or tension pressing on this area under the ribs, which is called the hypochondrium. This is a sign of congestion, mostly in the liver and gallbladder, which rule this area. As one continues over a period of weeks, this pain and tension will disappear and one's fingers will sink deeper under the ribs. This is quite important because it means that the liver's main function of governing the smooth dispersal of qi and blood is improving.

When the liver's coursing and discharging function is healthy, peristalsis is normal and digestion is good. Also, one's mood will be even and light and one will have regular elimination and freedom from depression. Therefore, one can see that just this first *hara shiatsu* move promoting the free flow of the liver-gallbladder qi can have a deeply healing effect.

Next, one positions their hands on their lower right abdomen next to their pelvic bone. With each exhalation, one presses down for a count of six. As one inhales, one moves up the abdomen until finally their hands are beneath the ribs again. One makes three passes up the abdomen on the right side. Anatomically this follows the course of the ascending colon.

Then, beginning at the solar plexus, one presses down the midline to just above the pubic bone. Likewise, one makes three other lines down the left abdomen moving from the center out to the sides. These passes down the left abdomen follow the course of the descending colon. One should repeat this entire sequence up the right and down the left sides of the abdomen three times, each time exerting a little more pressure.

Next, go back to any places where one felt special pain or resistance. As one exhales, exert pressure on these spots to the limits of one's tolerance but without torturing oneself. Often the same spots or areas will be sore day after day. But as one does this abdominal self-massage day by day, these areas will tend to become less sore and sensitive. Typically, in a relatively healthy person, after from two to four weeks of doing this regime daily, one's abdomen will be free from any such specially reactive areas.

This signals that incipient stagnations within the organs and bowels have been relieved even before they may have given rise to any other signs and symptoms.

According to some doctors, if one finds an actual lump or mass in the abdomen, besides having this checked by a primary health care professional, one should not press directly on the center of such a lump. Rather, one should search for a sore or sensitive spot on the edge or periphery of the mass. It is here that pressure should be exerted.[25]

Finally, one returns to the right hypochondrium and again presses once three times out to the right and then from the solar plexus once three times out to the left. This concludes one's daily session of abdominal self-massage.

After from two to four weeks of daily practice the average person will find their abdomen has become painless and supple. This should be accompanied by better bowel movements, better appetite, and therefore better, more abundant energy. This entire procedure takes approximately 15-20 minutes. It can be performed directly upon arising or just before bed. After the abdomen becomes pain free and normalized, one can do the massage every other or every few days. However, if one does not take care of oneself, after some time, the pain, lumps, and tension may return and these are signs that one's imbalance has also reestablished itself.

In traditional Japanese medicine, it is felt that sensitive spots, lumps, and tension in the abdomen are precursors to more serious disease. A person may otherwise be symptom free but to many Japanese physicians, if there is some abnormality in the

[25] Matsumoto, Kiiko, and Birch, Stephen, *Hara Diagnosis: Reflections on the Sea*, Paradigm Publications, Brookline, MA, 1988, p. 277-278

hara as diagnosed by palpation, there is some incipient disease process taking shape. Therefore, if one eliminates these abnormalities, one can abort such disease processes even before other signs and symptoms arise.

Also as stated above, nine of the eleven viscera and bowels of traditional Oriental medicine are located in and can be accessed through massage of the *hara*. Also, channels and network vessels connected to four of the most important viscera, the kidneys, spleen, stomach, and liver traverse the soft abdomen and are directly affected by this abdominal massage.

One cannot easily massage their entire body, but one *can* easily massage their abdomen. Since the abdomen or *hara* is the root of the entire body, massaging it massages the root of all the rest. If the roots of a plant are healthy, the leaves and branches will likewise tend to flourish. Although abdominal self-massage appears simple, it is based on voluminous and profound theory. For those interested in reading more about the *hara* and its importance in Oriental medicine and also more about *hara shiatsu*, the reader is referred to *Hara Diagnosis: Reflections on the Sea* by Matsumoto and Birch.[26]

Stress and Relaxation Therapy

In our culture stress is endemic — job stress, political stress, environmental pollution stress, relationship stress, sexual stress, travel stress, the stress of the constant decisions required by living in a "free" society. We have created a society which produces more stress than the human body can process and still remain healthy. Past a certain age, most of us will develop symptoms due to this fact. These symptoms may come and go and

---

[26] Ibid., p. 271-311

we can learn to keep them largely under control, but it is arrogant and unreasonable to think that we can forever keep up the often frenetic pace (physically or mentally) which many of us must (or believe we must) in order to survive and still be free of the ravages of stress.

Women especially find themselves at a time and place in history with "unlimited" options, where our roles are multiple and our sense of self often ill-defined. Our family structure is weaker and less supportive than at any time in American history; community support for parenting, women's health care, and menopausal issues is inadequate; divorce is endemic; and the stay-at-home mother-and-housewife is no longer an option for most of us. The arrival of menopause is another stressor in and of itself. It brings us face to face with aging, loss of fertility, and possibly the empty nest syndrome. We know that our culture is not supportive of postmenopausal women, and somewhere deep inside this may affect our sense of self worth. The constant demands on the time of the average 35-55 year old woman in our society often leave us with no "down" time and the feeling of being always behind, always pushed, always squeezed. This is what stagnation of qi, specifically liver qi, feels like.

The single most important part of any treatment program for symptoms related to qi stagnation is daily relaxation. We have already discussed the fact that the presence or absence of qi stagnation may spell the difference between the presence or absence of menopausal symptoms and/or their severity. This therapy, if done consistently and with perseverance, can make a difference on a long term basis, not only in terms of menopausal or other symptoms, but on the fundamental level of who a person is. The reason this therapy is so effective is that it addresses the long term effects of stress and emotional upset, which are at the root of all problems related to liver depression qi stagnation. In most cases having an emotional component, I believe this therapy can be as beneficial as good psychotherapy. This is because I believe that whatever happened that makes one frustrated or angry or bitter or afraid is better released and forgotten as quickly as possible. This does not mean that psychotherapy or other counseling may not also be useful in helping us sort out difficult situations in our lives, or that changes may not need to be made. However, regular daily relaxation will help us to let go of the things we cannot change and keep even the ones we can change in perspective so that external situations do not put our health in jeopardy.

The emotional responses that we have to situations are healthy in that they may help us to see that changes need to be made in our lives. Making changes to improve our life and limit our stress may be difficult. If our problems are complex, we may need the help of professional psychotherapists, our family, job counselors, our church, or friends. Perhaps for some women major changes are not possible. But no matter how we go about changing our lives or not changing them, holding onto anger and frustration is not useful and it has been demonstrated in both Western and Chinese medicine that it is deleterious to the health. Regular relaxation therapy will help us to do the letting go.

Daily relaxation therapy is one way to turn off the heat of stress, loosen the vise grip of that squeezed feeling, and lessen the toll that any pressures in our lifestyle can take on our health. In moments of anger and frustration, I find it useful to think of two things. First, consider whether what is making you angry will matter in a year. If not, then you may be wasting your precious energy being angry. Second, I try to remember that the best revenge is a good life. Stewing in my anger does not feel like a good life to me.

In order for this therapy to have measurable clinical effectiveness there are a few criteria which must be met.

1. It must result in somatic, physical relaxation as well as mental relaxation.

2. It must result in the center of consciousness coming out of one's head and into some part of the lower body, preferably the area of the lower abdomen.

3. It must be done a minimum of 20 minutes per day, although no longer than 30 minutes are required.

4. It must be done every day without missing a single day for at *least* 100 days.

There are many possible techniques which may accomplish this type of relaxation, including hatha-yoga, certain types of meditation, biofeedback training, etc. The easiest way that I have found, however, is to purchase one or two relaxation or stress reduction tapes available at health food stores, or "new age" bookstores. These take about 25-30 minutes each, are relatively inexpensive, and require minimal discipline.

Some people say that they cannot relax, or that it is very difficult for them to keep their mind concentrated during meditation, or that they do not have time to relax. It is precisely these people who need to relax the most. The tapes are helpful for these people in that, to some extent, they supply the needed concentration. Each time the mind wanders, the tape brings one back to the task at hand, so that one does not need to concentrate on anything, just to listen to the tape.

Additionally, it is best to try to do the tape at the same time each day, so that after a while it becomes like eating, getting dressed, or brushing your teeth, in other words a nondiscretionary part of your day.

At the end of three months a person may expect to be calmer, less flappable, and have a generally increased state of health with fewer of their prior symptoms manifesting.[27] At the end of three years of regular practice, one will be a different person altogether.

Flower therapy

People have been giving other people flowers for millennia to help them feel good. In Chinese medicine, there is actually a practice of flower therapy. Because the beauty of flowers bring most people joy and because joy is the antidote to the other four or six negative emotions of Chinese medicine,[28] flowers can help promote the free and easy flow of qi. It is said in Chinese medicine that, "Joy leads to relaxation (in the flow of qi)", and relaxation is exactly what the doctored ordered in case of menopausal syndrome. As Wu Shi-ji wrote in the Qing dynasty, "Enjoying flowers can divert a person from their boredom and alleviate suffering caused by the seven affects (or emotions)."

However, there is more to Chinese flower therapy than the beauty of flowers bringing joy. Flower therapy also includes aromatherapy. A number of Chinese medicinals come from plants which have flowers used in bouquets. For instance, Chrysanthemum flowers (*Ju Hua*, Flos Chrysanthemi Morifolii) are used to calm the liver and clear depressive heat rising to the upper body. The aroma of Chrysanthemum flowers thus also has a salutary, relaxing, and cooling effect on liver depression and

---

[27] Flaws, Bob, "Premenstrual Breast Distention", *Free & Easy, Traditional Chinese Gynecology for American Women*, Second Edition, Blue Poppy Press, Boulder, CO, 1986, p. 104

[28] In Chinese medicine, the emotions are sometimes counted as five and sometimes counted as seven. When counted as seven, fright and melancholy are added to anger, joy, thinking, sorrow, and fear.

depressive heat. Rose (*Mei Gui Hua*, Flos Rosae Rugosae) is used in Chinese medicine to move the qi and quicken the blood. Smelling the fragrance of Roses also does these same things. Other flowers used in Chinese medicine to calm the spirit and relieve stress and irritability are Lily, Narcissus, Lotus flowers, Orchids, and Jasmine. And further, taking a smell of a bouquet of flowers promotes deep breathing, and this, in turn, relieves pent up qi in the chest at the same time as it promotes the flow of qi downward via the lungs.

Light therapy

Light therapy, more specifically sunbathing or heliotherapy, is one of Chinese medicine's health preservation and longevity practices. Sunlight is considered the most essential yang qi in nature. Li Shi-zhen, the most famous Chinese doctors of the late Ming dynasty (1368-1644 CE) wrote, "*Tai yang* (literally, supreme yang but a name for the sun) is true fire." As he pointed out, "Without fire, heaven is not able to engender things, and without fire, people are not able to live." Because the back of the human body is yang (as compared to the front which is more yin), exposing the back to sunlight is a good way of increasing one's yang qi.

As we have seen above, most women's yang qi begins to decline by around 35 years of age. In women over 35 years of age, most premenstrual/perimenopausal fatigue, loose stools, lack of strength, poor memory, lack of concentration, poor coordination, decline in or lack of libido, low back and knee soreness and weakness, increased nighttime urination, and cold hands and feet are due to this decline first in the yang qi of the spleen and later in the yang qi of the spleen and kidneys. In addition, the spleen qi and kidney yang decline inevitably in both men and women as they get older. Therefore, a decline in the spleen and kidneys is a part of many older people's depression. In such cases,

95

sunbathing can help supplement the yang qi of the body, thereby strengthening the spleen and/or kidneys.

However, because the yang qi is also the motivating force which pushes the qi, increasing yang qi can also help resolve depression and move stagnation. Cao Ting-dong, a famous doctor of the Qing dynasty (1644-1911 CE) wrote:

> Sitting with the back exposed directly to the sun, the back may get warmed. This is able to make the entire body harmonious and smoothly flowing. The sun is the essence of *tai yang* and its light strengthens the yang qi of the human body.

In Chinese medicine, whenever the words harmonious and smoothly flowing are used together, they refer to the flow of qi and blood. Hence sun bathing can help course the liver and rectify the qi as well as fortify the spleen and invigorate the kidneys.

It has been said that sunlight is good for every disease except skin cancer. As we now know, overexposure to the sun can cause skin cancer due to sunlight damaging the cells of the skin. Therefore, one should be careful not to get too much sun and not to get burnt. In Chinese medicine, sun bathing should be done between the hours of 8-10 AM. One should only sun bathe between 11 AM-1 PM in winter in temperate, not tropical, latitudes. In addition, we believe that wearing a sun screen of SPF 15 or higher will not lessen the therapeutic warming effects of sun bathing from a Chinese medical point of view.

It is interesting to note that some Western researchers are coming to understand that exposure to light does play a role in many women's PMS as well as in seasonal affection depressive disorder (SADD).

Thread moxibustion

Thread moxibustion refers to burning extremely tiny cones or "threads" of aged Oriental mugwort directly on top of certain acupuncture points. When done correctly, this is a very simple and effective way of adding yang qi to the body without causing a burn or scar. Since most Western women with menopausal syndrome suffer from at least an element of spleen qi and possible kidney yang vacuity, adding yang qi to the body is a good idea in many perimenopausal women. However, if you suffer from depressive heat or yin vacuity, you should probably consult a professional practitioner before using this self-treatment.

To do thread moxa, one must first purchase the finest grade Japanese moxa wool. This is available from Oriental Medical Supply Co. (See below under magnet therapy for their address and phone number.) It is listed in their catalog under the name Gold Direct Moxa. Pinch off a very small amount of this loose moxa wool and roll it lightly between the thumb and forefinger. What you want to wind up with is a very loose, very thin thread of moxa smaller than a grain of rice. It is important that this thread not be too large or too tightly wrapped.

Next, rub a very thin film of Tiger Balm or Temple of Heaven Balm on the point to be moxaed. These are camphored Chinese medical salves which are widely available in North American health food stores or from Mayway Corp. whose address, telephone numbers, and fax numbers are given below in the next chapter. Be sure to apply nothing more than the thinnest film of salve. If such a Chinese medicated salve is not available, then wipe the point with a tiny amount of vegetable oil. Stand the thread of moxa up perpendicularly directly over the point to be moxaed. The oil or balm should provide enough stickiness to make the thread stand on end. Light the tread with a burning incense stick. As the thread burns down towards the skin, you will feel more and more heat. Immediately remove the burning thread when you begin to feel the burning thread go from hot to too hot. *Do not burn yourself.* It is better to pull the thread off too soon than too late. In this case, more is not better than enough. (If you do burn yourself, apply some *Ching Wan Hong* ointment. This is a Chinese burn salve which is available at Chinese apothecaries and from Mayway Corp. It is truly wonderful for treating all sorts of burns. It should be in every home's medicine cabinet.)

Having removed the burning thread and extinguished it between your two fingers, repeat this process again. To make this process go faster and more efficiently, one can roll a number of threads before starting the treatment. Each time the thread burns down close to the skin, pinch it off the skin and extinguish it *before* it starts to burn you. If you do this correctly, your skin will get red and hot to the touch but you will not raise a blister. Because everyone's skin is different, the first time you do this, only start out with three or four threads. Each day, increase this number until you reach nine to twelve threads per treatment.

This treatment is especially effective for women in their late 30s and throughout their 40s whose spleen and kidney yang qi has already become weak and insufficient or in older patients of both sexes. Since this treatment actually adds yang qi to the body, this type of thread moxa fortifies the spleen and invigorates the kidneys, warming yang and boosting the qi. Because the stimuli is not that strong at any given treatment, it must be done every day for a number of days. For women who suffer from perimeno-pausal fatigue, loose stools, cold hands and feet, low or no libido, and low back or knee pain accompanied by frequent nighttime urination which tends to be copious and clear, I recommend beginning this moxibustion just before ovulation, around day 10 in the cycle if you are still menstruating. It should then be repeated every day up through day one of the period and then suspended. It can be done for several months in a row, but should not usually be done continuously throughout the year, day in and day out. If your menses have completely stopped, you can begin this self-treatment any time.

There are three points which should be moxaed using this supplementing technique. These are:

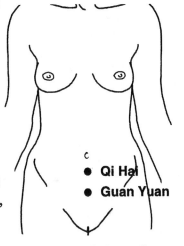

Qi Hai (Conception Vessel 6)

Guan Yuan (Conception Vessel 4)

Zu San Li (Stomach 36)

Qi Hai is located on the midline of the body, two finger widths below the navel. *Guan Yuan* is also located on the midline of the lower abdomen, four finger widths below the navel.

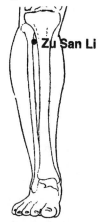

Zu San Li is located four finger widths below the lower edge of the kneecap between the tibia and fibula on the outside edge of the lower leg. However, we *highly* recommend visiting a local professional acupuncturist so that they can teach you how to do this technique safely and effectively and to show you how to locate these three points accurately.

In Chinese medicine, this technique is considered a longevity and health preservation technique. It is great for those people whose yang qi has already begun to decline due to the inevitable aging process. It should not be done by people with ascendant liver yang hyperactivity, liver fire, or depressive liver heat. It should also always be done starting from the topmost point and moving downward. This is to prevent leading heat to counterflow upward. If there is any doubt about whether this technique is appropriate for you, please see a professional practitioner for a diagnosis and individualized recommendation.

Magnet therapy

The Chinese have used magnet therapy since at least the Tang dynasty (618-907 CE). Placing magnets on the body is a safe and painless way of stimulating acupuncture points without inserting needles through the skin. Since magnets can be taped onto points and "worn" for days at a time, Chinese magnet therapy is able to provide easy, low cost, continuous treatment. It is also possible to tape on magnets at night and to wear them to bed. Special adhesive magnets for stimulating acupuncture points, such as Accu-Band Magnets, Corimag, or Epaule Patch TDK Magnets, may be purchased from:

Oriental Medical Supply Co.
1950 Washington St.
Braintree, MA 02184
Tel: (617) 331-3370 or 800-323-1839 Fax: (617) 335-5779

These magnets range in strength from 400-9,000 gauss, the unit measuring magnetic strength. For the treatments below, one can try 400-800 gauss magnets.

There is a set of four points called the Four Gates which are the four main points for treating liver depression qi stagnation. The Four Gates are comprised of two pairs of points. The first pair of points, *He Gu* (LI 4), is located on the top of the hand, between

the thumb and the index finger,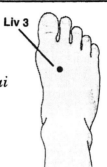
at the highest spot of the muscle when
the thumb and index finger are brought
close together. The second pair of points, *Tai
Chong* (Liv 3) is located on the top of
the foot, between the first and second
toes, about two inches away from the
margin of the web towards the body.

These points regulate the upbearing of the clear and
downbearing of the turbid, calm the mind and settle the spirit. In
my experience, all women with menopausal complaints suffer
from liver depression qi stagnation no matter what other Chinese
patterns they also exhibit. In fact, we can say that the degree of
severity of menopausal complaints is typically proportional to the
degree of severity of liver depression. Therefore, it is easy to see
why dealing with liver depression qi stagnation is so helpful for
the vaste majority of women with menopausal syndrome.

It isn't always necessary to treat all Four Gates and for some
people the sedative effect is too great if it's done this way. One
can reach dramatic results by treating these points contra
laterally, meaning, one point is done on the right side while the
other is done on the left. To treat the Four Gates with magnets,
one can tape a magnet with the south side down on *Tai Chong*,
and a magnet with its north side down on *He Gu*.

For women, the hand point (*He Gu*) should be on the right side
and the foot point (*Tai Chong*) on the left. According to Chinese
medicine left and right are a yin-yang pair. The left corresponds
to yang which is associated with the male element. The right
corresponds to yin and the female element.

Tai Chong can be combined in the same fashion with another
very helpful point, *Nei Guan* (Per 6).

101

This point is located on the inner side of the forearm between the two tendons. When used in combination, *Tai Chong* and *Nei Guan* rectifies the qi and resolves depression, loosens the chest and quiets the spirit. This combination of points is especially useful for chest oppression and rib-side pain, mental unrest, and insomnia. These two points are also best treated with magnets applied contra laterally according to the same principle for choosing left and right described above.

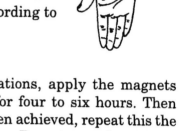

Per 6

For any of these two point combinations, apply the magnets during the day and leave in place for four to six hours. Then remove them. If good results have been achieved, repeat this the next day for the same length of time. Do not use these point combinations during sleep or late at night.

When insomnia is the main complaint in menopausal syndrome, magnets can also be used specifically at night to help you get to sleep. It is said in Chinese medicine that the ability to open and close the eyes has to do with the yang qi in two specific channels. These channels are called the *yin qiao mai* and the *yang qiao mai*. This translates as the yin and yang springing vessels. These two vessels both begin on the feet and meet at the eyes. The *yang qiao mai* carries yang qi upward to the head and specifically to the eyes. When this vessel is full of yang qi, the eyes are open and the person is awake. When this yang qi moves from the *yang qiao mai* into the *yin qiao mai* and is thence led back down into the lower and interior parts of the body, then the eyes close and one can go to sleep. Therefore, the yin and yang in the body that govern sleep and wake can be regulated by balancing the yin and yang qi in these two special vessels.

In most types of insomnia, yang qi is too full and is counter-flowing upward out of control. In order to promote sleep, yin must be nourished in order to "magnetize" or attract yang to move back downward and inward. In insomnia, the yang qi in the *yang qiao mai* is too full or replete, while the yin qi in the *yin qiao mai* is vacuous and insufficient. In order to re-establish the balance between yin and yang in these two vessels, one needs to drain the *yang qiao mai* and supplement the *yin qiao mai*. In acupuncture, this can be done by using gold needles to supplement the meeting point of the *yin qiao mai* and silver needles to drain the *yang qiao mai*. It is also possible to drain these points with copper and zinc needles respectively. However, this requires puncturing the skin and should only be done by a professional acupuncturist.

Happily, one can get the same effect by taping small magnets over these points. The meeting or command point of the *yin qiao mai* is called *Zhao Hai* (Ki 6). It is located one inch beneath the tip of the inner anklebone in a small depression below that bone. The meeting point of the *yang qiao mai* is called *Shen Mai* (Bl 62). It is located one inch below the tip of the outer anklebone, also in a small depression. In order to drain the yang qi from *Shen Mai*, tape a small body magnet south side down over this point just before bed at night. In order to supplement the yin qi at *Zhao Hai*, tape a small body magnet north side down over that point just before bed at night. Do this to both sets of points on both feet. Leave these magnets in place overnight, and remove them each morning when you wake. This can be done night after night until one is able to sleep without their aid.

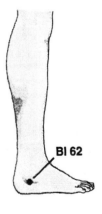

103

Chinese aromatherapy

In Chinese medicine, the qi is seen as a type of wind or vapor. The Chinese character for qi shows wind blowing over a rice field. In addition, smells are often referred to as a thing's qi. Therefore, there is a close relationship between smells carried through the air and the flow of qi in a person's body. Although aromatherapy has not been a major part of professionally practiced Chinese medicine for almost a thousand years, there is a simple aromatherapy treatment which one can do at home which can help alleviate premenstrual and perimenopausal irritability, depression, nervousness, anxiety, and insomnia.

In Chinese, *Chen Xiang* means "sinking fragrance." It is the name of Lignum Aquilariae Agallochae or Eaglewood. This is a frequent ingredient in Asian incense formulas. In Chinese medicine, Aquilaria is classified as a qi-rectifying medicinal. When used as a boiled decoction or "tea", Aquilaria moves the qi and stops pain, downbears upward counterflow and regulates the middle (*i.e.*, the spleen and stomach), and promotes the kidneys' grasping of the qi sent down by the lungs. I believe that the word sinking in this herb's name refers to this medicinal's down-bearing of upwardly counterflowing qi. Such upwardly counter-flowing eventually must accumulate in the heart, disturbing and causing restlessness of the heart spirit. When this medicinal wood is burnt and its smoke is inhaled as a medicinal incense, its downbearing and spirit-calming function is emphasized.

One can buy Aquilaria or *Chen Xiang* from Chinese herb stores in Chinatowns, Japantowns, or Koreatowns in major urban areas. One can also buy it from Chinese medical practitioners who have their own pharmacies. (See below for addresses, phone numbers, and fax numbers for companies selling Chinese herbs by mail.) It is best to use the powdered variety. However, powder may be made by putting a small piece of this aromatic wood in a coffee grinder. It is also ok to use small bits of the wood if powder is not available. Next one needs to buy a roll of incense charcoals. Place one charcoal in non-flammable dish and light it with a match. Then sprinkle a few pinches of Aquilaria powder on the lit charcoal. As the smoke rises, breathe in deeply. This can be done on a regular basis one or more times per day or on an as-needed basis by those suffering from restlessness, nervousness, anxiety, and irritability. For those who are experiencing depression, one can do this "treatment" on a regular basis at least three times per week.

This Chinese aromatherapy with Lignum Aquilariae Agallochae is very cheap and effective. I know of no side effects or contraindications.

Smoking and Recreational Drugs

We all know that smoking is deleterious to the health. From a Chinese medical point of view tobacco is dry and bitter and damages the lung qi. The lungs control the liver, as has been stated several times, and are responsible for astringing the surface to control perspiration which is very important for menopausal women. Furthermore, the lungs are the mother of the kidneys. If lung yin is damaged by the heat and dryness of tobacco, kidney yin will suffer. It is interesting to note here that smoking is a major risk factor for osteoporosis, and according to Chinese medicine, the kidney yin and essence nourish the bones and fill the marrow. Menopausal women can ill-afford to damage the kidney or lung yin.

Recreational drugs come in all types, and therefore have varying effects on the body. None of them, however, is useful for the menopausal woman. By and large they damage the liver and kidneys, leading to weakness of both these organs, the possible deleterious effects of which we have already discussed in detail from many points of view.

Finding Purpose and Meaning

In Western culture, as well as in China, up until fairly recently women did not often live into great age. Many women died in childbirth, from excessive childbearing or overwork, overexposure to the elements, and all manner of diseases. When we read the classics of Chinese medicine, we can see that a woman of 49 was considered an old woman.

In our century, at least in Western countries, this has changed. Most women have 15-30 good years after menopause in which to work, to contribute, to create. In fact, there may be fewer stressors on women during those years than there were in the previous two decades, as the duties of rearing children or producing income are lessened, leaving them freer to participate in other activities. At the same time, most women have, by popular media standards, lost much of their physical beauty and sexual attractiveness by this time in life. Women must find another source of self-esteem and life satisfaction than a good figure or a pretty face.

What I am leading up to here may be the most difficult self- help suggestion that I have, but it is perhaps the most important since it relates to our mind and heart. What I have observed is that the women for whom menopause is the easiest are those women with a purpose larger than themselves in their life. This purpose may be societal, political, ecological, artistic, or spiritual, but it must be strong enough to short circuit any media or other input from the popular cultural bias which damages basic self-esteem. By this I am not talking about some sort of false ego boosting. I am talking about usefulness which allows the development of inner strength and inner beauty. For, if we have not the impermanent beauty of youth nor the inner beauty which grows naturally from purpose and enthusiasm, it is then that our lives feel empty and mean, and there is room for anger, frustration, and depression. From a purely medical point of view, it is then that we feel stuck —and feeling stuck is the experience of liver depression/qi stagnation.

Of course this may not be easy and it may even sound trite, but among the people that I know, it is the ones with purpose who seem to be the healthiest. This is not to say that one has to be Mother Theresa, Indira Ghandi, or Jane Goodall to have a meaningful life. Neither is it to say that women with useful, purposeful lives have no health problems. Perhaps, however, if one feels useful, the magnitude of ones problems seem less, and are easier to cope with or rise above.

For some women this suggestion may imply volunteer work; for others it may imply a career change. There are no rules which say what gives meaning to a life. But it is certain that what gives meaning to life can change life for the better, bringing happiness and self-esteem in a real sense, which in turn cannot help but be reflected in the health of our bodymind.

Besides the suggestions in this chapter, there are other possible things that a woman can do for herself to help prevent the arising of disease. An important one that is not included in this chapter is proper diet. In fact, proper diet is so important that the following chapters is entirely devoted to it.

HELPING YOURSELF THROUGH DIET

There are people who believe that diet is the major key to health and that all health problems can be solved with a proper diet. After 20 years of work in the field of health care, I am convinced that this is not the case. While dietary advice should always be part of an overall health plan, it is my personal opinion that without proper exercise, no matter what we eat, it will not be digested as well or as completely as it could. Additionally, without proper relaxation, any tendency to stagnation will be aggravated, which also affects how well we digest our food and absorb nutrients. Nonetheless, our diet can make us sick, and major improvements in health can be made by adjustments in a person's diet. Especially diseases which have a digestive or eliminative component can be greatly affected by specific dietary adjustments.

For women who are perimenopausal, that is women who are nearing, in the middle of, or have just completed menopause, there are certain issues that diet can address and certain organs whose functions are important and can be supported through good diet. Obviously, the stomach, spleen, and intestines will be either positively or negatively affected by diet. This in turn will have an indirect but nonetheless important effect on the liver, kidneys, lungs, and heart. In fact, there is a lineage of Chinese medicine which came from a famous doctor, Li Dong-yuan (1180-

1251 C.E.), who based his entire treatment of the body and all its tissues and organs on rectifying the diet and digestion.[26]

Certainly there is solid Chinese medical theory to back up Dr. Li's ideas. If the spleen and stomach are healthy, there will be abundant qi and blood production with a concomitant increase in postnatal essence. This, in turn, will retard the aging process by supporting the kidneys and not requiring them to use up prenatal essence for basic metabolic processes. Also, an ample blood supply assures the heart and liver of adequate blood allowing them to house the spirit and ethereal soul comfortably. This ensures better sleep and emotional health. In fact, treatment of the spleen is an accepted method of treatment for liver disorders in general, even in acupuncture or herbal medicine.[27] Also, if the spleen is healthy, it will not draw excessively on the kidneys, which are the pilot light for the spleen/stomach which are, in turn, the "burner" responsible for the combustion of nutrients. Additionally, according to five phase theory, the spleen (earth) is the mother of the lungs (metal). Therefore, if earth is healthy, it can create metal, allowing the lungs to flourish. This then results both in good heart function and the natural control of the liver.

There are many foods and ways of eating food which support the health of the spleen/stomach. These include:

-eating mostly foods which are cooked and warm
-eating foods which are easily digestible

---

[26] Hsu, Hong-yen, and Preacher, William G., *Chen's History of Chinese Medical Science*, Oriental Healing Arts Institute, Long Beach, CA, 1977, p. 71

[27] Lee, Miriam, *Clinical Applications of St. 36, Sp. 6, Co. 4 and 11, and Lu. 7: One Combination of Points Can Treat Many Diseases*, self-published, Palo Alto, CA, p. 70

-eating mostly grains and vegetables with small amounts of meat and meat broths

-avoiding or limiting cold, frozen, and raw foods

-limiting foods which produce dampness, such as milk products, especially if there is a tendency to produce mucous

-using cautiously the warming spices such as ginger, cardamom, nutmeg, and cinnamon which benefit the digestion

Concerning cooked versus raw food, there has been a great deal of literature touting a raw foods diet as being the way to health. This is based on the presumption that raw foods have higher levels of vitamins and minerals which can be destroyed in cooking. However, while some cooking processes can be destructive to certain vital nutrients, what this idea fails to consider is how the digestive process actually works. Digestion is a process of combustion. The stomach must make everything that goes into it into 100 degree[28] soup before anything else can happen. Anything which helps the stomach by partially predigesting food, such as the process of cooking, will help the stomach do its job more efficiently and with less effort. This, in turn, allows the body to absorb the available nutrients more efficiently. Uncooked foods require more work from the stomach. Even lightly steaming or stir-frying aids the digestive process without harming most nutrients. Furthermore, if the nutrients which remain in cooked food are more absorbable than those in raw food, the net effect is improved nutrient absorption. Also, if the stomach does its job well the spleen, which is the next organ down the line in terms of digestion and energy production, will be more likely to do its job well. Consider further that one does not give raw foods to a sick person or to a baby, but rather cooked

---

[28] 100 degree here means 100 degrees Fahrenheit, not Centigrade.

foods which are more easily digestible, therefore imparting strength for recuperation or for growth.

The basic traditional diet that humans have thrived on for several millennia is a combination of cooked grains, whole, in noodles, or in breads, beans or legumes, vegetables (usually cooked) and fruits in season with small amounts of dairy and meat. Even modern weight loss diets such as the Pritikin program are based on this same combination. The reason that this diet works for weight loss is that it supports the spleen and stomach which automatically keep the body from accumulating dampness and phlegm, *i.e.*, fat.

Concerning dampness and phlegm, there are several foods which create dampness in the body —dairy products, excess meat, nuts, oils, and sugar. While small amounts will not cause problems in most people, when eaten to excess these can cause pathogenic accumulation of dampness. This in turn interferes with proper spleen function, decreasing the spleen's ability to transform phlegm and dampness, and to create enough qi and blood. This is a vicious circle which can lead to many other problems. For example, it is said that though the spleen is the creator of phlegm, the lungs are its home. This means that phlegm may lodge in the lungs leading to upper respiratory dysfunction. Phlegm may obstruct the channels, where it may cause numbness, paralysis, lumps, nodules, or tumors. Finally it may obstruct the heart where it disturbs the spirit, causing behavioral changes, madness, or unconsciousness. Dampness, which is a slightly different entity from a technical Chinese medical point of view, can cause stiffness of the joints, sluggish movement, heavy limbs, fuzzy thought processes, or turbid, cloudy, sticky secretions or excretions. Considering all the problems that pathogenic dampness or phlegm can cause, foods that contribute to their accumulation should be limited.

Concerning the caveat against chilled foods and frozen drinks, these are even harder for the stomach/spleen to process and are rather like dousing a precious fire with ice water. Again remember that the stomach must bring all foods up to body temperature before they can be digested and you can see how much harder it is for frozen and cold foods to be digested. Also we must consider that, up until 40-50 years ago, there was no refrigeration and frozen foods[29] did not really exist. While refrigeration is a great gift for keeping food fresher longer, it is questionable whether or not we should eat foods straight out of the freezer or refrigerator. Any food will be easier to digest at room temperature. As for ice water, it tastes great on a hot day, but should probably be drunk between meals so as not to slow down digestion thereby leading to stagnant food and/or dampness.

The mild warming spices, most of the basic pumpkin pie spices if you noticed, give a mild boost to the movement of qi and slightly invigorate the stomach without the damage that can be done by strong qi movers such as caffeine and heavy pungent spices such as cayenne pepper and jalapenos. These are fine to include in the diet in judicious amounts as long as they do not aggravate heat symptoms such as hot flashes or night sweats.

While the liver is more deeply affected by emotions than by diet, there are foods which can aggravate an imbalanced liver, and should be avoided. These include:

   -coffee including decaff, and other caffeinated foods or
      beverages

---

[29] Frozen foods here mean foods which are eaten frozen or chilled, such as ice cream and frozen yogurt. It does not mean foods which have been frozen for storage and then cooked. Although not as healthy as fresh food, frozen foods which are then cooked before eating are ok.

113

-alcohol, except in small, infrequent amounts
-greasy, fried, or oily foods
-spicy, pungent, hot dishes such as curries or chilies
-excessive meat consumption and other hard to digest
    foods such as nuts and beans
-chemicals, pollutants, and preservatives

Lets go over these one by one. Caffeine, especially in the form of coffee (and even decaff), is not a food according to Chinese medicine. It is used as a drug, and in small doses. Its functions are to strongly activate the qi and bring the energy from the core of the body to the surface. The activity of qi has to do with the consumption of yin by yang. Therefore, by strongly activating the qi, a certain amount of yin and blood (substance and fluid) will be used up. This exhaustion of yin and blood skews the relationship between yin and yang which in menopausal women is already precarious at best. The net effect of long term caffeine consumption is, therefore, extremely deleterious to a woman's health most especially at this time in her life. Of course, if a woman suffers from any symptoms of liver qi stagnation, she will really like the kick which the caffeine gives to the qi and may have a terrible time overcoming the habit. While the caffeine temporarily frees up the movement of the qi, it will eventually waste the blood. Since the liver blood is what allows its qi to flow unobstructedly, the entire situation is actually exacerbated in the long run. If a woman can make only one change in her diet, slowly weaning herself from coffee (including decaff) and other forms of caffeine is probably the best dietary change that she can make for her health.

Alcohol in small amounts from time to time relaxes the mind and makes for social conviviality. Its energetic nature is, however, damp and hot. When used to excess it overheats the liver and stomach, and dampens the spleen. Since dampness weakens the spleen and excess heat injures the blood and exacerbates any tendency to heat symptoms, we can see that neither of the attributes of alcohol is useful for a menopausal woman. In short, one should keep their consumption to an occasional beer or glass of wine.

In addition to dampening the spleen, greasy or oily foods tend to clog the digestive mechanism. Their frequent consumption can lead to food stagnation and spleen dampness. Also, it is the liver/gallbladder which is responsible for the metabolism of fats through the creation and secretion of bile. Over-consumption of these foods creates excessive work for the liver, which, like an engine running for too long, will tend to become overheated.

Spicy foods have a similar effect to that of caffeine. Most of us with liver stagnation will be drawn to them as they give a kick to the liver qi. However, because the acrid or pungent flavor relates to the metal phase according to five phase theory, its excessive consumption will tend to weaken the lungs, whose job it is to keep the liver in check. Additionally, since foods with this flavor tend to be hot and dry in nature, they typically overheat the liver and stomach and dry the blood. In any disease which has an element of qi stagnation, the consumption of acrid or pungent foods is classically forbidden.[30]

This book does not tout vegetarianism. Although meat need only be eaten in small amounts or in the form of broths, it is probably important for most people to include a small amount of it in their diets, because it is an excellent food for preventing qi and blood emptiness. On the other hand, large quantities of it are difficult to digest, produce pathogenic dampness, and are unnecessary for adequate protein consumption. Soups made from meat broths or

---

[30] Wolfe, Honora, *The Breast Connection: A Laywoman's Guide to the Treatment of Breast Disease by Chinese Medicine*, Blue Poppy Press, Boulder, CO, 1989. p. 74

marrow bones are an excellent way to get the most nourishment from meat without the part which is hard to digest and unnecessary for health.

The effects on our food supply of preservatives and other chemicals or pollutants found in the soil and water is known to be deleterious to the health. Many of these substances are carcinogenic or toxic to various organs. While it may not always be possible to buy organically grown food, it is advisable to do so as much as possible. Especially as we get older, our bodies are less able to neutralize or excrete these substances and it is advisable to eliminate them as much as possible from our diet. Also, by demanding more organically grown foods we are sending a message to the retailers, the food growers, and to the government bodies with which they interact. This will eventually have the effect of increasing support for organic farming methods. As the supply of organic foods increases, the prices of these foods will come down.

Finally, this discussion has spoken of the effect of diet on other viscera leaving out the kidneys. While the kidneys are affected by the health of all the other viscera and bowels, it is also possible to treat the kidneys directly through diet. It is said in the *Ling Shu (Spiritual Pivot)*, Chapter 36 that "the essence extracted from the five cereals reaches the bones and nourishes the brain and marrow." Since bones, marrow, and brain tissue are the outgrowth or flourishing of the kidney essence, this passage is referring to the nourishment of the kidneys. By using the term five cereals there are two implications. One is that all the five flavors of five phase theory will have an effect on the kidneys, and that the consumption of grains specifically is supplementing to the body in general.

In classical Chinese dietary theory, grains should be partially processed or polished which makes them easier to digest. This is interesting in light of the fact that, according to Western

116

nutritional biochemistry, excess bran and fiber from grains creates an excess of phytic acid in the body inhibiting the absorption of calcium and other minerals into the bones, again bringing us back to the kidney essence.

Other foods which are specifically good for the kidneys are soups made from marrow bones, walnuts, lotus seeds, grapes, pork and turtle meat, chicken, actual kidney meat from sheep or ox, potatoes, and pears.

If liver yang is hyperactive with heat symptoms in the upper body, foods which lower yang include barley, beef broth, asparagus, apples, bananas, lettuce, and celery.

Foods which calm the spirit include rice, oyster, longan fruit, wheat and wheat germ, and many types of mushrooms.

From this discussion, it is easy to see why diet and nutrition is so important for maintaining good health and especially when the body is going through the delicate balancing act of menopause. Below are a selection of Chinese medicinal teas and porridges. These are made by combining Chinese herbs with other common foods. This is where Chinese herbal medicine and Chinese dietary therapy blend into each other.

Chinese Medicinal Porridges

Chinese medicinal porridges are a specialized part of Chinese dietary therapy. Because porridges are already in the form of 100° soup, they are a particularly good way of eating otherwise nutritious but nevertheless hard-to-digest grains. When Chinese medicinals are cooked along with those grains, one has a high-powered but easily assimilable "health food" of the first order.

For liver depression qi stagnation, cook 50g of white rice with 10g of Pericarpium Citri Reticulatae Viride (*Qing Pi*). Eat this one time per day. Another possibility is to cook 5g of Flos Pruni (*i.e.*, plum flowers) with 100g of white rice with enough water to make a thin porridge or gruel.

For spleen qi vacuity with pronounced fatigue, cook 30g of Radix Astragali Membranacei (*Huang Qi*) with 6g of Pericarpium Citri Reticulatae (*Chen Pi*) in 600ml of water for 20 minutes. Remove the dregs and then use the resulting medicinal "tea" to cook 50g of white rice. Another possibility for treating spleen qi vacuity fatigue and lack of strength is to take 3g of powdered Radix Panacis Ginseng (*Ren Shen*) and cook this with 100g of white rice in water. Yet another option is to take 5g of ginseng and 20g of powdered Sclerotium Poriae Cocos (*Fu Ling*) and cook this with 60g of white rice in water. During the last 5-7 minutes of cooking, add a couple of slices of fresh ginger. If you cannot find ginseng, you can use 30g of Radix Codonopsitis Pilosulae (*Dang Shen*) cooked with 50g of white rice in water. Remove the codonopsis at the end and eat the resulting porridge.

For heart blood-spleen qi vacuity depression, insomnia, poor memory, and/or heart palpitations, cook 100g of white rice with 50g of Semen Coicis Lachryma-jobi (*Yi Yi Ren*) and 10 red dates (Fructus Zizyphi Jujubae, *Da Zao*). Or cook 100g of white rice in chicken broth plus 10 red dates and eat this for dinner every evening for a number of days.

For insomnia and anxiety due to blood and yin vacuity, use 15g of either Semen Biota Orientalis (*Bai Zi Ren*) or Semen Ziziphi Spinosae (*Suan Zao Ren*) with 100g of white rice and again cook with enough water to make a thin porridge or gruel. Or simply eat cream of wheat every evening before bed instead of dessert.

118

For depression accompanied by phlegm confounding or blocking the orifices of the heart, try cooking 5g of powdered Rhizoma Acori Graminei (*Shi Chang Pu*) with 50g of white rice in water.

For heart palpitations, one can try taking 15g of Fluoritum (*Zi Shi Ying*) and boiling this in 300ml of water down to 150ml. Then remove the dregs and use this liquid to cook 100g of glutinous or so-called, sticky or sweet rice. Add a little brown sugar to taste and eat this morning and evening on an empty stomach.

To supplement the kidneys and fills the essence, one can first cook into porridge 100g of regular white rice or brown rice if you prefer. During the last 5 minutes of cooking the rice, add three slices of fresh ginger. After the rice is cooked, take out the ginger slices, powder 20g of Gelatinum Cornu Cervi (*Lu Jiao Jiao*), and mix this into the rice porridge. Eat this every day for 3-5 days. However, because this formula supplements kidney yang, do not use this porridge unless you have symptoms of kidney yang vacuity, *i.e.*, cold feet, frequent urination, night-time urination, low back pain, *and* decreased libido.

For numerous other Chinese medicinal porridge formulas for all sorts of complaints, see Bob Flaws's *The Book of Jook: Chinese Medicinal Porridges: A Healthy Alternative to the Typical Western Breakfast* also published by Blue Poppy Press.

Chinese Medicinal Tas

Chinese medicinal teas consist of using only one or two Chinese herbal medicinals in order to make a tea which is then drunk as one's beverage throughout the day. Such Chinese medicinal teas are usually easier to make and better tasting than multi-ingredient, professionally prescribed decoctions. They can be used as an adjunct to professional prescribed Chinese herbs or as an adjunct to acupuncture or other Chinese therapies for depression.

119

For liver depression qi stagnation, take 100-150g of fresh plums and add to 320ml of water in a pot and boil for three minutes. Then add 2g of green tea and 25g of honey and steep for 10 minutes. Take one dose in the morning and another dose in the evening. This formula is especially effective for abdominal distention and epigastric oppression associated with liver depression. Another easy tea for liver depression qi stagnation can be made by boiling 25g each of Fructus Immaturus Citri Aurantii (*Zhi Shi*) and Pericarpium Citri Reticulatae (*Chen Pi*), *i.e.*, orange peel, in water for several minutes. Then add 2g of green tea and steep for 10 minutes. Drink the resulting tea as a beverage any time during the day. Yet another tea for liver depression qi stagnation may be made by taking 10g of Tuber Curcumae (*Yu Jin*), *i.e.*, turmeric, and boiling it in one liter of water with 5g of Radix Glycyrrhizae (*Gan Cao*), *i.e.*, licorice. Then add 2g of green tea and a little honey to taste. Drink this as a beverage throughout the day.

For liver depression/depressive heat, boil 30g each of green tea and Fructus Gardeniae Jasminoidis (*Shan Zhi Zi*) in one quart of water and boil until the liquid is reduced by half. Remove the dregs and drink one cup of this liquid in the morning and another in the evening. Or one can take 15g of Flos Chrysanthemi Morifolii (*Ju Hua*) and steep this with 2g of green tea in boiling water for 10 minutes. Then drink the resulting tea as a beverage throughout the day. In addition, jasmine tea purchased at Asian specialty food shops is a good background beverage for those with liver depression with or without heat.

For spleen vacuity fatigue and lack of strength, boil 8g of Radix Panacis Ginseng (*Ren Shen*) for an hour or more in eight ounces of water. Drink this as a tea throughout the day. Asian specialty food stores often sell small porcelain ginseng cookers. These are lidded cups meant to be placed in a pan of water to create a small double-cooker. Basically, the longer you cook ginseng, the more you get out of it. As a substitute for ginseng, you can use double the amount of Radix Codonopsitis Pilosulae (*Dang Shen*). *Do not use ginseng if you suffer from hypertension or high blood pressure.*

If you suffer from spleen qi and heart blood vacuity, you can try making a tea from 9g of Radix Pseudostellariae (*Tai Zi Shen*), and 15g of Semen Levis Tritici Aestivi (*Fu Xiao Mai*). Place both of these ingredients in a thermos and steep in boiling water for 20 minutes. Then drink as a tea throughout the day. Or you can use 5-10 pieces of Arillus Euphoriae Longanae (*Long Yan Rou*). Place these dried fruits in a double boiler or pressure cooker and steam thoroughly. Then put them in a teacup and steep in boiling water for 10 minutes. Drink the resulting liquid as a tea. Yet another possibility is to boil 10 pieces of Fructus Zizyphi Jujubae (*Da Zao*) in water until the fruit are thoroughly cooked (*i.e.*, completely soft). Then use the resulting liquid to steep 5g of green tea. Drink this as a tea any time throughout the day.

For insomnia due to heart yin and blood vacuity, grind 15g of Semen Biotae Orientalis (*Bai Zi Ren*) into pieces. Boil with water for 10 minutes and add honey to taste. Drink either before or after dinner. Or boil 15g of Fructus Mori Albi (*Sang Zhen*) in water. Remove the dregs and drink one packet per day. Another option is to grind into powder equal amounts of Fructus Schisandrae Chinensis (*Wu Wei Zi*) and Fructus Lycii Chinensis (*Gou Qi Zi*). Then use 5g of this powder steeped in boiling water for 10 minutes as a tea throughout the day. Or you may use 9g of Semen Zizyphi Spinosae (*Suan Zao Ren*). Pound these into pieces, steep in boiling water for 10 minutes, and drink throughout the day.

For phlegm obstruction with liver depression/depressive heat, grind Rhizoma Acori Graminei (*Shi Chang Pu*), 6g, Flos Jasmini (*Mo Li Hua*), 6g, and green tea, 10g, into coarse powder. Soak some of this powder in boiling water and drink as a tea any time of the day. (You can also use jasmine tea bought at an Asian specialty food shop.) Another formula for phlegm obstruction

121

disturbing the heart spirit but without the heat consists of Dens Draconis (*Long Chi*), 10g, and Rhizoma Acori Graminei (*Shi Chang Pu*), 3g. First boil the Dens Draconis in water for 10 minutes. Then add the Rhizoma Acori Graminei and continue boiling for another 10-15 minutes. Remove the dregs and drink any time of the day, 1-2 packets per day. The doses given are for a one day's supply.

For fire disturbing the heart spirit characterized by restlessness and insomnia, vexation and agitation, a red tongue tip, sores on the tip of the tongue, and heart palpitations, one can boil 60g each of Medulla Junci Effusi (*Deng Xin Cao*) and Folium Lophatheri Gracilis (*Dan Zhu Ye*). Remove the dregs and drink the resulting tea warm at any time of the day, one packet per day.

For excessive menstrual bleeding or functional uterine bleeding due to spleen-kidney dual vacuity, one can make a tea out of Semen Nelumbinis Nuciferae (*Lian Zi*), 5g, and tea leaves, 30g. Soak the tea leaves in boiling water. Then reserve the tea and discard the dregs. Soak the lotus seeds in warm water for a few hours. Then stew them with a little sugar. Add the tea water and stir well. Once again remove the dregs and drink the remaining liquid as a tea throughout the day.

If excessive menstruation or functional uterine bleeding is due to heat forcing the blood to move frenetically or recklessly outside its pathways, one can take Herba Artemisiae Apiaceae (*Qing Hao*), 6g, and Cortex Radicis Moutan (*Dan Pi*), 6g. Wash these two ingredients and place them along with 3g of tea leaves in a teacup. Cover them with boiling water and allow to steep for 15-20 minutes. Discard the dregs, add a little sugar to taste, and drink frequently throughout the day.

Yet another simple Chinese herbal tea to stop excessive vaginal bleeding due to heat is to take Herba Cephalanoploris Segeti

(*Xiao Ji*), 10g, and steep in boiling water. Drink the resulting liquid as a beverage throughout the day.

And finally, for depression alternating with agitation, one can use Fructus Levis Tritici Aestivi (*Fu Xiao Mai*), 30g, Fructus Zizyphi Jujubae (*Da Zao*), 10 pieces, and mix-fried Radix Glycyrrhizae (*Gan Cao*), 6g. Boil these three ingredients in water, strain the liquid, and drink this frequently as tea.

For more information on Chinese medicinal teas, see Zong Xiao-fan and Gary Liscum's *Chinese Medicinal Teas: Simple, Proven, Folk Formulas for Common Diseases & Promoting Health* also published by Blue Poppy Press.

The medicinals in all the formulas in this chapter can be purchased by mail from:

China Herb Co.
165 W. Queen Lane
Philadelphia, PA 19144
Tel: 215-843-5864
Fax: 215-849-3338
Orders: 800-221-4372

Mayway Corp.
1338 Mandela Parkway
Oakland, CA 94607
Tel: 510-208-3113
Orders: 800-2-Mayway
Fax: 510-208-3069
Orders by fax: 800-909-2828

Nuherbs Co.
3820 Penniman Ave.
Oakland, CA 94619
Tel: 510-534-4372
Orders: 800-233-4307
Fax: 510-534-4384
Orders by fax: 800-550-1928

PROFESSIONALLY ADMINISTERED THERAPIES: PREVENTIVE & REMEDIAL

Self-care is an essential part of any comprehensive health care plan. Indeed, it may be the largest and most important part. There are times, however, when it is appropriate and necessary to seek out the support of professional health care providers. The reasons may be either preventive, remedial, or both. If you are a menopausal woman with symptoms that are more than a slight annoyance, it is probably wise to seek out professional care. Estrogen replacement therapy (ERT) is the most common therapy given to menopausal women by Western medical practitioners and for some women it is no doubt appropriate. (See chapter 11 for a more complete discussion.) Chinese and other more natural medicines offer other remedial and preventive options for symptomatic and asymptomatic menopausal women which may be preferable for many.

If you are menopausal and taking estrogen replacement therapy (ERT) but would like to stop, Chinese herbal medicine may be able to help you. If you are in your late 30s or early 40s and have any menstrual irregularity, PMS symptoms, fibrocystic breasts, excessive bleeding, or cramps, not only can Chinese herbal medicine and acupuncture help you with your current problems, but by doing so may help you have an easier, less symptomatic menopause. If you are a woman who has passed menopause, who is not on ERT, is planning to stop ERT, or would like to stop ERT, there are other options to keep your bones strong, maintain cardiovascular health, and/or to deal with other potential health problems.

In this chapter we discuss the two main professionally administered Chinese medical therapies which may be of special help to menopausal women. These are acupuncture, and Chinese herbal medicine.

Acupuncture

Acupuncture is the best known of the various methods of treatment which go to make up Chinese medicine. When the average Westerner thinks of Chinese medicine, they probably first think of acupuncture. In China, acupuncture is actually a secondary treatment modality. Most Chinese immediately think of herbal medicine when they think of Chinese medicine. Nevertheless, many menopausal complaints responds very well to correctly prescribed and administered acupuncture.

What is acupuncture?

Acupuncture primarily means the insertion of extremely thin, sterilized, stainless steel needles into specific points on the body where practitioners of Chinese medicine have known for centuries there are special concentrations of qi and blood. Therefore, these points are like switches or circuit breakers for regulating and balancing the flow of qi and blood over the channel and network system we described above.

As we have seen, menopausal syndrome typically contains a key component of liver depression qi stagnation. Secondarily, many menopausal complaints are symptoms of erroneously counterflowing qi—in other words, qi which is moving in the wrong direction. Since acupuncture's forte is the regulation and rectification of the flow of qi, it is an especially good treatment mode for correcting liver depression qi stagnation and symptoms of erroneously counterflowing qi. In that case, insertion of acupuncture needles at various points in the body moves stagnant qi in the liver and leads the qi to flow in its proper directions and amounts.

As a generic term, acupuncture also includes several other methods of stimulating acupuncture points, thus regulating the flow of qi in the body. The main other modality is moxibustion. This means the warming of acupuncture points mainly by burning dried, aged Oriental mugwort on, near, or over acupuncture points. The purpose of this warming treatment are to 1) even more strongly stimulate the flow of qi and blood, 2) add warmth to areas of the body which are too cold, and 3) add yang qi to the body to supplement a yang qi deficiency. Other acupuncture modalities are to apply suction cups over points, to massage the points, to prick the points to allow a drop or two of blood to exit, to apply Chinese medicinals to the points, to apply magnets to the points, and to stimulate the points by either electricity or laser.

What is a typical acupuncture treatment like?

In China, acupuncture treatments are given every day or every other day, three to five times per week depending on the nature and severity of the condition. In the West however, health care delivery differs greatly from China, making it financially unfeasible for most patients to receive as many treatments per week. Western patients suffering from menopausal complaints typically respond very well to acupuncture treatment performed twice a week for the first few weeks, following up with treatment every week for another several weeks. After that, a maintenance course of monthly sessions is highly recommended, since liver depression tends to be a recurrent condition. In severe, stubborn cases, acupuncture treatment may have to continue for several months. In general, one can expect their improvement from acupuncture to be gradual and progressive. Based on my clinical experience, if acupuncture is combined with diet and life-style changes, Chinese herbs, and a selection of the self-care treatments recommended above the results will be even quicker and the relief of symptoms even more complete.

When the person comes for their appointment, the practitioner will ask them what their main symptoms are, will typically look at their tongue and its fur, and will feel the pulses at the radial arteries on both wrists. Then, they will ask the patient to lie down on a treatment table and may palpate their abdomen and the zones traversed by the different channels to feel for areas of constriction, tenderness, and blockage. Based on the patient's pattern discrimination, the practitioner will select anywhere from one to eight or nine points to be needled.

The needles used today are ethylene oxide gas sterilized disposable needles. This means that they are used one time and then thrown away, just like a hypodermic syringe in a doctor's office. However, unlike relatively fat hypodermic needles, acupuncture needles are hardly thicker than a strand of hair. The skin over the point is disinfected with alcohol and the needle is quickly and deftly inserted somewhere typically between one quarter and a half inch. In some few cases, a needle may be inserted deeper than that, but most needles are only inserted relatively shallowly.

After the needle has broken the skin, the acupuncturist will usually manipulate the needle in various ways until he or she feels that the qi has "arrived." This refers to a subtle but very real feeling of resistance around the needle. When the qi arrives, the patient will usually feel a mild, dull soreness around the needle, a slight electrical feeling, a heavy feeling, or a numb or tingly feeling. All these mean that the needle has tapped the qi and that treatment will be effective. Once the qi has been tapped, then the practitioner may further adjust the qi flow by manipulating the needle in certain ways, may simply leave the needle in place, usually for 10-20 minutes, or may attach the needle to an electro-acupuncture machine in order to stimulate

128

the point with very mild and gentle electricity. After this, the needles are withdrawn and thrown away. *Thus there is absolutely no chance for infection from another patient.*

Does acupuncture hurt?

In Chinese, it is said that acupuncture is *bu tong*, painless. However, most patients will feel slight sensations of soreness, heaviness, electrical tingling, or distention. When done well and sensitively, it should not be sharp, biting, burning, or really painful. If there is any discomfort at all, it should be negligible.

How quickly will I feel the result?

One of the best things about the acupuncture treatment of menopausal complaints is that its effects are often immediate. Since many of the mechanisms of menopausal syndrome have to do with stuck qi, as soon as the qi is made to flow, the symptoms disappear. Therefore, many patients begin to feel better after the very first treatment.

In addition, because irritability and nervous tension are also mostly due to liver depression qi stagnation, most people will feel an immediate relief of these symptoms while still on the table. Typically, one will feel a pronounced tranquility and relaxation within five to ten minutes of the insertion of the needles. Many patients do drop off to sleep for a few minutes while the needles are in place.

Who should get acupuncture?

Since most professional practitioners in the West are legally entitled to practice under various acupuncture laws, most acupuncturists will routinely do acupuncture on every patient. Since acupuncture's effects on liver depression qi stagnation are usually relatively immediate, this is usually a good thing for sufferers of this commonly encountered pattern of disharmony.

When a woman's menopausal complaints mostly have to do with qi vacuity, blood vacuity, or yin vacuity, then acupuncture is most effective when combined with internally administered Chinese herbal medicinals. Although moxibustion can add yang qi to the body, acupuncture needles cannot add qi, blood, or yin to a body in short supply of these. The best acupuncture can do in these cases is to stimulate the various viscera and bowels which engender and transform the qi, blood, and yin. Chinese herbs, on the other hand, can directly introduce qi, blood, and yin into the body, thus supplementing vacuities and insufficiencies of these. In cases of menopausal syndrome, where qi, blood, and yin vacuities are pronounced, as is typically the case, one should use acupuncture in combination with Chinese medicinals.

Ear acupuncture

Acupuncturists believe there is a map of the entire body in the ear and that by stimulating the corresponding points in the ear, one can remedy those areas and functions of the body. Therefore, many acupuncturists will not only needle points on the body at large but also select one or more points on the ear. In terms of menopausal complaints, needling the point *Shen Men* (Spirit Gate) can have a profound effect on relaxing tension and irritability and also improving sleep. There are also other points, such as the Sympathetic Point, the Brain Point, and the Subcortex Point which can be very effective in the treatment of the emotional discomfort, depression, restlessness, and anxiety associated with many women's menopausal syndrome.

The nice thing about ear acupuncture points is that one can use tiny "press needles" which are shaped like miniature thumb-tacks. These are pressed into the points, covered with adhesive tape, and left in place for five to seven days. This method can

130

provide continuous treatment between regularly scheduled office visits. Thus ear acupuncture is a nice way of extending the duration of an acupuncture treatment. In addition, these ear points can also be stimulated with small metal pellets, radish seeds, or tiny magnets, thus getting the benefits of stimulating these points without having to insert actual needles.

Chinese Herbal Medicine

Chinese herbal medicine is one of the most effective natural methods of treating menopausal complaints or preventing their arisal. Studies on the effectiveness of herbal medicine for treating menopausal women for a variety of symptoms are written about in Traditional Chinese Medical journals on a regular basis. Typical amelioration rates of these studies are in the 80-95% range. In professionally practiced Chinese medicine, herbs are rarely used singly. Most formulas, whether prepared as a powder, pill, tincture, or tea are a combination of from six to twenty herbs.

Herbs are effective in cases of vacuity because they can actually add qi, blood, yin, and/or yang to the body. Furthermore, herbs work largely through the medium of the blood and yin, unlike acupuncture which mostly manipulates qi. Since most meno- pausal health issues relate to the blood and yin and to insufficiency or vacuity, herbs are often an appropriate choice. Herbs have the added advantage of being whole and biochemically complex substances made up of a balance of various synergistic chemical parts and hormone precursors. This means that they are easier for the body to utilize than single, synthesized drugs, and that in turn means they are less likely to cause side effects.

However, such freedom from side effects is based on correct administration in turn based on a correct professional diagnosis.

131

This is why it is usually a good idea not to self-medicate. Do not make the mistake of thinking that since herbal medicines are natural substances, herbs are completely benign. The wrong herbs or the wrong dosage can make a person sick or worsen their health.

So if you are seriously interested in taking herbs for preventive or remedial menopausal care, it is wise to seek professional assistance in choosing the appropriate formulas.

Experimenting with Chinese patent medicines

In reality, qualified professional practitioners of Chinese medicine are not yet found in every North American community. In addition, some people may want to try to heal their menopausal complaints as much on their own as possible. More and more health food stores are stocking a variety of ready-made Chinese formulas in pill and powder form. These ready-made, over-the-counter Chinese medicines are often referred to as Chinese patent medicines. Although my best recommendation is for readers to seek Chinese herbal treatment from professional practitioners, below are some suggestions of how one might experiment with Chinese patent medicines to treat the main perimenopausal complaints.

In chapter 6, I have given the signs and symptoms of main Chinese patterns associated with most women's menopausal syndrome. These are:

1. Liver blood, kidney yin vacuity
2. Ascendant liver yang hyperactivity
3. Spleen-kidney yang vacuity
4. Accumulation of phlegm & stagnation of qi
5. Heart blood, spleen qi vacuity

6. Heart yin & blood vacuity
7. Heart & kidneys not interacting
8. Kidney yin & yang dual vacuity
9. Liver depression qi stagnation

If the reader can identify their main pattern from chapter 6, then there are some Chinese patent remedies that they might consider trying.

Xiao Yao Wan (also spelled *Hsiao Yao Wan*)

Xiao Yao Wan is one of the most common Chinese herbal formulas prescribed. Its Chinese name has been translated as Free & Easy Pills, Rambling Pills, Relaxed Wanderer Pills, and several other versions of this same idea of promoting a freer and smoother, more relaxed flow. As a patent medicine, this formula comes as pills, and there are both Chinese-made and American-made versions of this formula available over the counter in the North American marketplace.[31]

The ingredients in this formula are:

Radix Bupleuri (*Chai Hu*)
Radix Angelicae Sinensis (*Dang Gui*)
Radix Albus Paeoniae Lactiflorae (*Bai Shao*)
Rhizoma Atractylodis Macrocephalae (*Bai Zhu*)
Sclerotium Poriae Cocos (*Fu Ling*)
mix-fried Radix Glycyrrhizae (*Gan Cao*)
Herba Menthae Haplocalycis (*Bo He*)
uncooked Rhizoma Zingiberis (*Sheng Jiang*)

---

[31] When marketed as a dried, powdered extract, this formula is sold under the name of Bupleurum & Tang-kuei Formula.

This formula treats the pattern of liver depression qi stagnation complicated by blood vacuity and spleen weakness with possible dampness as well. Bupleurum courses the liver and rectifies the qi. It is aided in this by Herba Menthae Haplocalycis or mint Dang Gui and Radix Albus Paeoniae Lactiflorae or white peony nourish the blood and soften and harmonize the liver. Rhizoma Atractylodis Macrocephalae or atractylodes and Sclerotium Poriae Cocos or poria fortify the spleen and eliminate dampness. Mix-fried licorice aid these two in fortifying the spleen and supplementing the liver, while uncooked ginger aids in both promoting and regulating the qi flow and eliminating dampness.

When menopausal complaints are accompanied by the signs and symptoms of liver depression, spleen qi vacuity, and an element of blood vacuity, one can try taking this formula. However, after taking these pills at the dose recommended on the packaging, if one notices any side effects, then stop immediately and seek a professional consultation. Such side effects from this formula might include nervousness, irritability, a dry mouth and increased thirst, and red, dry eyes. Such side effects show that this formula, at least without modification, is not right for you. At least one of the ingredients, Radix Bupleuri (*Chai Hu*) is very drying and can damage yin. Although the formula may be doing you some good, it is also causing some harm. Remember, Chinese medicine is meant to cure without side effects, and as long as the prescription matches one's pattern there will not be any.

This formula can be taken in combination with other, more supplementing and moistening formulas.

Dan Zhi Xiao Yao Wan

Dan Zhi Xiao Yao Wan or Moutan & Gardenia Rambling Pills is a modification of the above formula which also comes as a patent medicine in the form of pills.[32] It is meant to treat the pattern of liver depression transforming into heat with spleen vacuity and possible blood vacuity and/or dampness. The ingredients in this formula are the same as above except that two other herbs are added:

Cortex Radicis Moutan (*Dan Pi*)
Fructus Gardeniae Jasminoidis (*Shan Zhi Zi*)

These two ingredients clear heat and resolve depression. In addition, Cortex Radicis Moutan or moutan quickens the blood and dispels stasis and is good at clearing heat specifically from the blood. Some Chinese doctors say to take out uncooked ginger and mint, while other leave these two ingredients in.

Basically, the signs and symptoms of the pattern for which this formula is designed are the same as those for *Xiao Yao Wan* above plus signs and symptoms of depressive heat. These might include a reddish tongue with slightly yellow fur, a bowstring and rapid pulse, a bitter taste in the mouth, and increased irritability.

This formula has the same drawbacks as its parent prescription of being relatively drying. It too can be combined with other, more supplementing and moistening formulas.

Chai Hu Jia Long Gu Mu Li Wan

Chai Hu Jia Long Gu Mu Li Wan or Bupleurum, Dragon Bone & Oyster Shell Pills are the pill form of a formula which has been used in China and other Asian countries for 1,700 years. It is for the treatment of liver depression/depressive heat and spleen vacuity

---

[32] When marketed as a dried, powdered extract, this formula is called Bupleurum & Peony Formula.

135

causing mental-emotional anxiety, unrest, insomnia, and heart palpitations. Its ingredients include:

Radix Bupleuri (*Chai Hu*)
Radix Panacis Ginseng (*Ren Shen*)
Rhizoma Pinelliae Ternatae (*Ban Xia*)
Sclerotium Poriae Cocos (*Fu Ling*)
Ramulus Cinnamomi Cassiae (*Gui Zhi*)
Radix Scutellariae Baicalensis (*Huang Qin*)
Fructus Zizyphi Jujubae (*Da Zao*)
Os Draconis (*Long Gu*)
Concha Ostreae (*Mu Li*)
dry Rhizoma Zingiberis (*Gan Jiang*)
Radix Et Rhizoma Rhei (*Da Huang*)

Because this formula contains rhubarb, this formula is especially effective for those suffering from constipation. If this formula causes diarrhea, its use should be immediately discontinued and professional advice sought.

Er Chen Wan

Er Chen Wan means Two Aged (Ingredients) Pills.[33] This is because, two of its main ingredients are aged before using. This formula is used to transform phlegm and eliminate dampness. It can be added to many other formulas when phlegm dampness complicate the pattern. Its ingredients include:

Rhizoma Pinelliae Ternatae (*Ban Xia*)
Sclerotium Poriae Cocos (*Fu Ling*)
mix-fried Radix Glycyrrhizae (*Gan Cao*)
Pericarpium Citri Reticulatae (*Chen Pi*)

---

[33] When sold as a dried, powdered extract, this formula is called Citrus & Pinellia Combination.

uncooked Rhizoma Zingiberis (*Sheng Jiang*)

Liu Wei Di Huang Wan

This formula, whose name means Six Flavors Rehmannia Pills, nourishes liver blood and kidney yin. It is the primary formula to treat symptoms of yin vacuity. It can be combined with other patent medicines when there is a strong component of yin vacuity. Its ingredients are:

cooked Radix Rehmanniae (*Shu Di*)
Fructus Corni Officinalis (*Shan Zhu Yu*)
Radix Dioscoreae Oppositae (*Shan Yao*)
Rhizoma Alismatis (*Ze Xie*)
Sclerotium Poriae Cocos (*Fu Ling*)
Cortex Radicis Moutan (*Dan Pi*)

If there are signs and symptoms of vacuity heat, then another formula should be used instead. It is made by adding two more ingredients to the above:

Rhizoma Anemarrhenae Aspheloidis (*Zhi Mu*)
Cortex Phellodendri (*Huang Bai*)

This is then called *Zhi Bai Di Huang Wan*, Anemarrhena & Phellodendron Rehmannia Pills. For instance, a very commonly prescribed combination is *Zhi Bai Di Huang Wan* and *Bu Zhong Yi Qi Wan* described below for spleen qi vacuity, liver depression, kidney yin vacuity, and yin vacuity and/or damp heat.

137

Jin Gui Shen Qi Wan

The name of these commonly available Chinese patent pills translates as Golden Cabinet Kidney Qi Pills. The golden cabinet is an allusion to the name of the book this formula is first recorded in, the *Jin Gui Yao Lue (Essentials from the Golden Cabinet)* dating from 200-250 CE. This is the most famous formula for the treatment of kidney yang vacuity, and it can be combined with other formulas when kidney yang vacuity complicates a patient's pattern discrimination. Its ingredients include:

cooked Radix Rehmanniae (*Shu Di*)
Fructus Corni Officinalis (*Shan Zhu Yu*)
Radix Dioscoreae Oppositae (*Shan Yao*)
Sclerotium Poriae Cocos (*Fu Ling*)
Rhizoma Alismatis (*Ze Xie*)
Cortex Radicis Moutan (*Dan Pi*)
Radix Lateralis Praeparatus Aconiti Carmichaeli (*Fu Zi*)
Cortex Cinnamomi Cassiae (*Rou Gui*)

Because this formula contains at least two very hot herbs, one should not take this formula if they have any signs or symptoms of heat or they should get a diagnosis and prescription for this formula from a professional practitioner.

Tian Wang Bu Xin Dan

The name of this formula translates as Heavenly Emperor's Supplement the Heart Elixir.[34] This formula comes as a Chinese patent medicine in pill form. It treats insomnia, restlessness, fatigue, and heart palpitations due to yin, blood, and qi vacuity,

---

[34] When marketed as a desiccated, powdered extract, this formula is sold under the name Ginseng and Zizyphus Formula.

with an emphasis on heart yin and liver blood vacuity. Its ingredients include:

uncooked Radix Rehmanniae (*Sheng Di*)
Radix Scrophulariae Ningpoensis (*Xuan Shen*)
Fructus Schisandrae Chinensis (*Wu Wei Zi*)
Tuber Asparagi Cochinensis (*Tian Men Dong*)
Tuber Ophiopogonis Japonici (*Mai Men Dong*)
Radix Angelicae Sinensis (*Dang Gui*)
Semen Biotae Orientalis (*Bai Zi Ren*)
Semen Zizyphi Spinosae (*Suan Zao Ren*)
Radix Salviae Miltiorrhizae (*Dan Shen*)
Radix Polygalae Tenuifoliae (*Yuan Zhi*)
Sclerotium Poriae Cocos (*Fu Ling*)
Radix Codonopsitis Pilosulae (*Dang Shen*)

Bai Zi Yang Xin Wan
(also spelled *Pai Tsu Yang Hsin Wan*)

The name of this formula translates as Biota Seed Nourish the Heart Pills. This is another commonly used over-the-counter Chinese patent pill. It is usually marketed for insomnia characterized by heart yin and liver blood vacuity complicated by an element of phlegm obstruction. Its ingredients include:

Semen Biotae Orientalis (*Bai Zi Ren*)
Fructus Lycii Chinensis (*Gou Qi Zi*)
Radix Scrophulariae Ningpoensis (*Xuan Shen*)
uncooked Radix Rehmanniae (*Sheng Di*)
Tuber Ophiopogonis Japonici (*Mai Men Dong*)
Radix Angelicae Sinensis (*Dang Gui*)
Sclerotium Poriae Cocos (*Fu Ling*)
Rhizoma Acori Graminei (*Shi Chang Pu*)
Radix Glycyrrhizae (*Gan Cao*)

139

Tabellae *Suan Zao Ren Tang*

This is the tableted form of a famous spirit-calming Chinese medicinal decoction, Zizyphus Spinosa Decoction. Its ingredients are:

Semen Zizyphi Spinosae (*Suan Zao Ren*)
Radix Ligustici Wallichii (*Chuan Xiong*)
Sclerotium Poriae Cocos (*Fu Ling*)
Rhizoma Anemarrhenae Aspheloidis (*Zhi Mu*)
Radix Glycyrrhizae (*Gan Cao*)

This formula is for insomnia and restlessness or anxiety due primarily to liver blood vacuity with possibly a little heat disturbing the heart spirit.

Ding Xin Wan

The name of this Chinese patent pill translates as Stabilize the Heart Pills. It supplements the heart qi and blood, quiets the heart spirit, and clears heat disturbing the heart from the liver and/or stomach. It can be taken when there is heart qi and blood vacuity with transformative heat leading to restless spirit, anxiety, heart palpitations, and insomnia. Its ingredients include:

Radix Codonopsitis Pilosulae (*Dang Shen*)
Radix Angelicae Sinensis (*Dang Gui*)
Sclerotium Pararadicis Poriae Cocos (*Fu Shen*)
Radix Polygalae Tenuifoliae (*Yuan Zhi*)
Semen Zizyphi Spinosae (*Suan Zao Ren*)
Semen Biotae Orientalis (*Bai Zi Ren*)
Radix Scutellariae Baicalensis (*Huang Qin*)
Tuber Ophiopogonis Japonici (*Mai Men Dong*)
Succinum (*Hu Po*)

An Mian Pian

These are called Quiet Sleep Pills. They can be used by themselves or combined with other appropriate patent pills for insomnia and restlessness due to liver depression transforming heat and liver blood not nourishing the heart spirit. Their ingredients are:

Semen Zizyphi Spinosae (*Suan Zao Ren*)
Radix Polygalae Tenuifoliae (*Yuan Zhi*)
Sclerotium Poriae Cocos (*Fu Ling*)
Fructus Gardeniae Jasminoidis (*Shan Zhi Zi*)
Massa Medica Fermentata (*Shen Qu*)
Radix Glycyrrhizae (*Gan Cao*)

Tong Jing Wan (also spelled To Jing Wan)

The name of these pills means Painful Menstruation Pills. Because of the relationship between the qi and the blood, menopausal complaints are often complicated by blood stasis even though the pattern of blood stasis is typically not listed as a pattern of menopausal syndrome. If there is either enduring qi stagnation or enduring blood and yin vacuity, this may give rise to static blood, remembering that synonyms for static blood include dead blood and dry blood. The symptoms of blood stasis include painful menstruation with the passage of dark clots, pain which is stabbing or intense in nature and tends to be fixed in position, a dark, dusky facial complexion, possible black circles under the eyes, purplish lips, a purplish tongue, possible static blood patches or dots on the tongue, spider nevi, small, red hemangiomas, varicosities, hemorrhoids, or thrombophlebitis, and a bowstring, choppy pulse.[35] In such cases, this pill can be taken along with other appropriate

---

[35] A choppy pulse is a fine, somewhat slow pulse which tends to speed up and slow down (often with the breathing) but does not necessarily skip any beats.

formulas when blood stasis is an important factor in someone's pattern. Its ingredients are:

Tuber Curcumae (*Yu Jin*)
Rhizoma Sparganii (*San Leng*)
Radix Rubrus Paeoniae Lactiflorae (*Chi Shao*)
Radix Angelicae Sinensis (*Dang Gui*)
Radix Ligustici Wallichii (*Chuan Xiong*)
Radix Salviae Miltiorrhizae (*Dan Shen*)
Flos Carthami Tinctorii (*Hong Hua*)

Xue Fu Zhu Yu Wan

The name of these pills means Blood Mansion Dispel Stasis Pills. They are yet another Chinese patent medicine in pill form for the treatment of blood stasis. Its ingredients include:

Semen Pruni Persicae (*Tao Ren*)
Radix Angelicae Sinensis (*Dang Gui*)
Flos Carthami Tinctorii (*Hong Hua*)
uncooked Radix Rehmanniae (*Sheng Di*)
Radix Achyranthis Bidentatae (*Niu Xi*)
Radix Ligustici Wallichii (*Chuan Xiong*)
Radix Rubrus Paeoniae Lactiflorae (*Chi Shao*)
Fructus Citri Aurantii (*Zhi Ke*)
Radix Bupleuri (*Chai Hu*)
Radix Platycodi Grandiflori (*Jie Geng*)
Radix Glycyrrhizae (*Gan Cao*)

Bu Zhong Yi Qi Wan

The name of this formula translates as Supplement the Center & Boost the Qi Decoction. It strongly supplements spleen vacuity. It is commonly used to treat central qi fall, *i.e.*, prolapse of the stomach, uterus, or rectum due to spleen qi vacuity. However, it is a very complex formula with a very wide range of indications. It supplements the spleen but also courses the liver and rectifies the qi. It is one of the most commonly prescribed of all Chinese herbal formulas and these pills can be combined with a number of others when spleen qi vacuity and liver depression play a significant role in someone's menopausal symptoms, however without significant blood vacuity or particular dampness. Its ingredients are:

Radix Astragali Membranacei (*Huang Qi*)
Radix Panacis Ginseng (*Ren Shen*)
Radix Glycyrrhizae (*Gan Cao*)
Rhizoma Atractylodis Macrocephalae (*Bai Zhu*)
Radix Angelicae Sinensis (*Dang Gui*)
Pericarpium Citri Reticulatae (*Chen Pi*)
Rhizoma Cimicifugae (*Sheng Ma*)
Radix Bupleuri (*Chai Hu*)
Rhizoma Atractylodis Macrocephalae (*Bai Zhu*)

Da Bu Yin Wan

The name of this standard prescription translates as Greatly Supplementing Yin Pills. It is a commonly used formula for severe yin vacuity with vacuity heat. Its ingredients include:

cooked Radix Rehmanniae (*Shu Di*)
Plastrum Testudinis (*Gui Ban*)
Rhizoma Anemarrhenae Aspheloidis (*Zhi Mu*)
Cortex Phellodendri (*Huang Bai*)

This pill can be combined with others when one wants to enrich yin and clear vacuity heat even more forcefully.

143

Zuo Gui Wan

These pills are called Restore the Left (Kidney) Pills. They are also a very strong yin-enriching, blood-supplementing pre-scription. Their ingredients are:

cooked Radix Rehmanniae (*Shu Di*)
Radix Dioscoreae Oppositae (*Shan Yao*)
Fructus Corni Officinalis (*Shan Zhu Yu*)
Semen Cuscutae Chinensis (*Tu Si Zi*)
Fructus Lycii Chinensis (*Gou Qi Zi*)
Radix Achyranthis Bidentatae (*Niu Xi*)

Gan Mai Da Zao Wan

This is a pill form of a very simple yet very effective formula. It consists of:

Fructus Levis Tritici Aestivi (*Fu Xiao Mai*)
mix-fried Radix Glycyrrhizae (*Gan Cao*)
Fructus Zizyphi Jujubae (*Da Zao*)
Bulbus Lilii (*Bai He*)
Cortex Albizziae Julibrissin (*He Huan Pi*)
Radix Polygoni Multiflori (*He Shou Wu*)
Sclerotium Poriae Cocos (*Fu Ling*)

This formula can be added to other if there are yin vacuity night sweats or when there is emotional depression, anxiety, heart palpitations, and insomnia.

Du Huo Sheng Ji Wan

This is a famous formula for low back and joint pain due to a combination of liver-kidney yin and yang vacuity with wind, damp, cold impediment obstructing the free flow of the channels and network vessels. It can be used for the treatment of low back pain associated with osteoporosis. Its ingredients include:

Radix Angelicae Pubescentis (*Du Huo*)
Cortex Eucommiae Ulmoidis (*Du Zhong*)
Ramulus Loranthi Seu Visci (*Sang Ji Sheng*)
Radix Codonopsitis Pilosulae (*Dang Shen*)
cooked Radix Rehmanniae (*Shu Di*)
dry Rhizoma Zingiberis (*Gan Jiang*)
Sclerotium Poriae Cocos (*Fu Ling*)
Cortex Cinnamomi Cassiae (*Rou Gui*)
Radix Angelicae Sinensis (*Dang Gui*)
Radix Glycyrrhizae (*Gan Cao*)

Ge Jie Da Bu Wan

These last are also a very effective formula for treating osteoporosis due to liver-kidney yin and yang vacuity. They are called Gecko Greatly Supplementing Pills because A) they contain gecko lizard as an ingredient, and B) they supplement yin and yang, qi and blood altogether. In addition, they contain ingredients which specifically strengthen the low back and the fortify the sinews and bones. Their ingredients include:

Gecko (*Ge Jie*)
Radix Codonopsitis Pilosulae (*Dang Shen*)
Radix Astragali Membranacei (*Huang Qi*)
Fructus Lycii Chinensis (*Gou Qi Qi*)
Radix Angelicae Sinensis (*Dang Gui*)
Sclerotium Poriae Cocos (*Fu Ling*)

145

cooked Radix Rehmanniae (*Shu Di*)
Fructus Ligustri Lucidi (*Nu Zhen Zi*)
Radix Glycyrrhizae (*Gan Cao*)
Radix Dioscoreae Oppositae (*Shan Yao*)
Fructus Chaenomelis Lagenariae (*Mu Gua*)
Rhizoma Cobotii Barometsis (*Gou Ji*)
Radix Morindae Officinalis (*Ba Ji Tian*)
Rhizoma Atractylodis Macrocephalae (*Bai Zhu*)
Radix Dipsaci (*Xu Duan*)
Cortex Eucommiae Ulmoidis (*Du Zhong*)
Rhizoma Polygonati (*Huang Jing*)
Rhizoma Drynariae (*Gu Sui Bu*)

The above are only the most famous and commonly used formulas which are currently available over the counter at American health food stores and at Asian specialty food stores in Asian communities in North America. They can be ordered by phone, fax, or mail from:

Mayway Corp.
1338 Mandela Parkway
Oakland, CA 94607
Tel. 510-208-3113
Orders: 1-800-2-Mayway
Fax: 510-208-3069 Orders by fax: 1-800-909-2828

This company is one of the largest importers and distributors of Chinese herbs and Chinese herbal products in North America and Europe. They have a very nice, easy to use catalog with easy ordering numbers so you do not need to worry about pronouncing the Chinese names of these formulas.

There are many other important formulas used in the professional practice of Chinese medicine. However, for these, you will need to see your local professional practitioner. If you experiment with Chinese herbal patent medicines for your menopausal complaints, please be careful. Be sure to follow the six guideposts for assessing the safety of any medications you take.

Six guideposts for assessing any over-the-counter medication

In general, you can tell if *any* medication and treatment are good for you by checking the following six guideposts:

1. Digestion
2. Elimination
3. Energy level

4. Mood
5. Appetite
6. Sleep

If a medication, be it modern Western or traditional Chinese, gets rid of your symptoms and all six of these basic areas of human health improve, then that medicine or treatment is probably OK. However, even if a treatment or medication takes away your major complaint, *if it causes deterioration in any one of these six basic parameters,* then that treatment or medication is probably not OK and is certainly not OK for long-term use. When medicines and treatments, even so-called natural, herbal medications, are prescribed based on a person's pattern of disharmony, then there is healing without side effects. According to Chinese medicine, this is the only kind of true healing.

ESTROGEN REPLACEMENT THERAPY: PROS & CONS

History of ERT/HRT Use

Despite recent revelations about potential long term risks, the most common therapy given to menopausal women in developed nations is estrogen or hormone replacement therapy (ERT/HRT). This therapy involves oral, cutaneous patch, or vaginal cream administration of estrogen to replace what the ovaries have stopped producing. Usually oral estrogen is given in combination with some form of synthetic progesterone for at least part of the month to minimize some of the possible side effects of unopposed estrogen therapy such as increased risk of endometrial growths or cancer. This combination of medications prolongs the youthful hormonal state of women well past their reproductive years.

HRT has gone through many changes in the last several decades. In the West, estrogen replacement therapy was first used in the 1920s for women who has lost their ovaries. It became quite fashionable in the early 60s for menopausal women to take estrogen and the sales quadrupled over the next 10 years. By the early 70s as many as 22 million prescriptions per year for estrogen therapy were being written for menopausal and post menopausal women.[36] Women were told they would age more slowly, look better, and avoid the discom-

---

36   Shoemaker, E.S., Forney, J.P., and MacDonald, P.C., "Estrogen Treatment of Postmenopausal Women: Benefits and Risks", *Journal of the American Medical Association*, #238, Jan., 1977, p. 1524

forts of menopause at the same time. Also, the drug companies have had a lot to gain by touting estrogen therapy as a larger proportion of our population reaches middle age.

However, by the mid 70s, research began to appear linking estrogen use with increased rates of endometrial or uterine cancer. At that point the use of estrogen therapy dropped rapidly for several years. However, once it was discovered that the use of synthetic progesterone in combination with estrogen taken for at least part of the month seemed to lower this risk, the use of HRT therapy grew to even higher levels in the 1980s and 90s. Progesterone allows the uterine lining to be shed at the end of each month much like a small menstrual period, preventing a build up of the uterine lining that can lead to uterine cancer.

ERT/HRT Therapy or Not?

While this therapy is still a popular one, questions about its long term risks have not all been answered and recent research is far less positive. Although adding progestin to the estrogen cycle reduces the risk of uterine cancer, some studies have linked synthetic progestin, like the progesterone in birth control pills, to an increased risk of high blood pressure, heart disease, high LDL cholesterol, and stroke.[37] Other studies indicate exactly the opposite, that the use of ERT which includes progestin for part of the month greatly reduce the risk of hardening of the arteries, high cholesterol, and heart disease.[38] Still other doctors state that ERT combined with progestin, calcium, and sodium fluoride could be used safely for the prevention of osteo-

---

[37] Greenwood, Sadja, *op.cit.*, p. 90

[38] "Report on Menopause", ABC network television, *20/20*, August 10, 1990

porosis in most women.[39] Clearly, despite the enthusiasm that some doctors still show for HRT, there are many unanswered questions about these drugs.

It is a fact that HRT can prevent many of the physical discomforts which may arise during menopause, such as hot flashes, night sweats, vaginal dryness or atrophy, as well as possibly preventing or slowing osteoporosis. Its effects on cardiovascular health are still unclear at this point. What neither ERT nor HRT will do is prevent wrinkles or outward signs of aging, nor will it help deal with the existential or psychosocial issues which menopause often brings to the surface.

While proponents of HRT therapy still believe that its use will increase life span by preventing hip and spinal fractures and cardiovascular disease, recent research challenges these claims and there are other drawbacks to HRT therapy that have always been known. Side effects may include breast distention or soreness, weight gain or water retention and edema, headaches, or mild to severe nausea. Severe side effects may include an increased risk for gallstones and gallbladder disease. Moreover, while studies linking the use of ERT/HRT to breast cancer are still conflicting, most doctors will not prescribe it for women who have had breast cancer or who are at a high risk for that disease.

HRT is also not prescribed for women with clinical depression, uterine fibroids, diabetes, thrombophlebitis or other thromboembolic disorders, serious migraines, or known gallbladder disease. Also, some doctors will not prescribe HRT for women who are overweight, since women who are more than 25-30 pounds overweight are at a higher risk for uterine/endometrial cancer due to the fact that natural estrogen is formed in body fat tissue, and higher levels of blood estrogen have been linked to increased incidence of both breast and uterine cancer.

---

[39]   Gambrell Jr., Don R., *op.cit.*, p. 23

Finally, while some women feel much better on HRT, others dislike having a monthly "period." Still others find the increased visits to the doctor which HRT demands to be a financial strain. It is also true that increased visits to the doctor often result in more medical tests, more drugs, possibly even more surgeries.

New Estrogen Research!

Before deciding whether or not to take estrogen, women should also know that there is recent evidence suggesting that the most common form of estrogen used in Western HRT therapy is linked to higher rates of breast cancer, while an alternative form of HRT is actually linked to lower rates of breast cancer.[40]

There are three forms of estrogen that are active in the female body: estrone, estradiol, and estriol. Estradiol is the primary estrogen produced by the ovaries, and estrone is formed by conversion of estradiol. Estrone is thought to be the estrogen primarily responsible for facilitating carcinoma of the breast. Estriol is produced in large amounts during pregnancy and is proven to be protective against breast cancer. High levels of estriol are found in vegetarian and Asian women, both of whom have much less risk of breast cancer.

Unfortunately, the most popular form of estrogen replacement in menopausal women is conjugated estrogens such as *Premarin*® which, in the intestinal tract, are converted mostly to estrone, the hormone that has been implicated in breast cancer. While studies looking at the effects of oral estrogen replacement of this type have found only a slight increase in breast cancer risk, it would seem more sensible to take an alternative form of estrogen that actually can help prevent breast cancer if such were available.

---

[40] Whitaker, Julian, MD, "Preventing Breast Cancer", *Health & Healing: Tomorrow's Medicine Today*, January, 1994

Estriol, which is not used in most estrogen replacement therapy in the West, was shown to inhibit breast cancer in mice 25 years ago.[41] This form of estrogen is not converted to estrone in the intestines and seems to block the stimulatory effect of estrone on breast tissue. A study directed by H.M. Lemon, MD done in 1966, showed that women with breast cancer have a reduced urinary excretion rate of estriol, while women without breast cancer have higher levels of estriol compared with estrone and estradiol.[42]

While this hormone is commonly used in Europe, the FDA has refused to approve its use in the U.S. It is, however, available through a few physicians. One doctor in Washington state has been using estriol with his patients for over a decade. He has found that by adding small amounts of estrone and estradiol to large amounts of estriol, he can rapidly alleviate the symptoms of menopause and secure the benefits that all three estrogens provide against osteoporosis without the fear of facilitating breast cancer. He calls this compound "tri-estrogen" and he combines it with a natural progesterone (not *Provera*®, which is a synthetic progestin) to prevent the potential problems connected with unopposed use of estrogen replacement while lessening the potential side effects of progestins such as high blood pressure and stroke.[43]

Estriol can be gotten in U.S. through a few pharmacies and physicians. You can contact the following pharmacies which make the above "tri-estrogen" and ask them for a referral to a doctor in your area through whom you may be able to get a prescription:

---

[41] *Ibid.*, p. 3

[42] Lemon, H.M., MD, "Reduced Estriol Excretion in Patients with Breast Cancer Prior to Endocrine Therapy", *Journal of the American Medical Association*, 1966, 196: 1128-1134.

[43] *Ibid.*, p. 3

College Pharmacy in Colorado Springs, CO (800) 888-9358

Women's International Pharmacy in Madison, WI
(800) 279-5708 or (608) 221-7800

ApotheCure in Dallas, TX (800) 969-6601

For more detail on all these subjects, I suggest you read *The Estrogen Alternative* by Raquel Martin, published by Healing Arts Press. Ms. Martin's book includes extensive lists of sources for many types of natural hormones.

The Chinese Medical View of HRT

Let me begin this discussion of the Chinese medical view of HRT by saying that Chinese doctors had isolated sex hormones from urine by 125 BCE and used these hormones as rejuvenating supplements. Such medicines were called autumn mineral and autumn dew water.[44] Therefore, there is nothing "un-Chinese medicine" about HRT *per se*. In fact, HRT in a somewhat more primitive form has been a part of Chinese medicine for more than 2,000 years.

However, from the Chinese medical point of view, ERT, with or without progestins, may have some definite drawbacks in some patients. When looking at the potential side effects of HRT, one can see that they are similar to those of the birth control pill. This is not unusual, since both drugs contain estrogen and, in most cases, both contain progestin or synthetic progesterone as well. According to Chinese medicine, the way that the birth control pill causes infertility is by causing an excessive supplementation of yin and body fluids which then results in qi stagnation and blood stasis in the pelvis. Therefore, depending on the woman, we may suppose that HRT can do the same thing.

Consider that unopposed estrogen can lead to uterine growths or exacerbate uterine fibroids both of which, according to

---

[44]   Robert Temple, *The Genius of China: 3,000 Years of Science, Discovery, and Invention*, Simon & Schuster, NY, 1989, p. 127-131

Chinese medicine, usually include blood stasis as part of their diagnosis. Blood stasis can cause a number of problems, the most immediate one being qi stagnation (see chart on p.44), since the qi and blood flow together, and stagnation of one will, over time, lead to stagnation of the other. Since the smooth flow of qi and blood is largely controlled by the liver, this stagnation and stasis mostly affects the liver, at least at first. Liver depression/qi stagnation and its consequences have been discussed at some length in chapter four, but lets look at the possible side effects of HRT in this light.

Breast pain and distention are the first side effect listed. In Chinese medicine, this symptom is a classic one due to liver depression/qi stagnation and consequent heat and congested qi blocking the channels and vessels which traverse the breast tissue. Nausea as a result of ERT/HRT is caused by a combination of dampness encumbering the spleen and liver qi invading the stomach which leads to the stomach qi counterflowing upward instead of downbearing (*i.e.*, descending) as it normally should. Edema or water retention is likewise due to damp accumulation further aggravating liver depression. The headaches associated with HRT are yet again a combination of dampness and liver depression. Gallbladder disease is usually related to damp heat in the liver and gallbladder plus liver qi congestion and, sometimes, blood stasis as well.

It is interesting also to note that many of the disorders which contraindicate the use of HRT, breast or uterine cancers, thromboembolic diseases, serious high blood pressure, severe migraines, uterine fibroids, stroke, and liver/gallbladder diseases, all typically involve either liver depression/qi stagnation, blood stasis, or both. If HRT over a long period of time has a negative impact on these disorders, it is a logical hypothesis that HRT may contribute to liver depression/qi stagnation and to blood stasis.

Some women have no side effects on HRT. In those women, we must assume that HRT supplements yin without causing damp

155

repletion which in turn obstructs the free flow of qi and blood. In these women, HRT may be a perfectly safe and effective therapy which is simple to use and relatively inexpensive. However, when HRT does result in symptoms of damp accumulation, qi stagnation, and blood stasis, then its use is unwarranted, since, from the Chinese medical point of view, the only true healing is healing without side effects.

So the issue is not whether HRT is good or bad. The issue is that HRT is not good for every woman. For those women in whom HRT causes side effects, whether short or long term, Chinese medicine provides equally inexpensive, equally effective therapies which, when correctly prescribed are completely without side effects since they fit the individual woman's unique bodily needs. In fact, treatment given on the basis of an individualized pattern discrimination improves the health of the entire organism since it helps bring the whole organism back into a state of dynamic balance.

Chinese Herbal Alternatives

Let us look a little more closely at progesterone by itself in relationship to Chinese medical theory. Progesterone is clearly a yang qi supplement both for the kidneys and the spleen. I say this because conditions which modern Western medicine says are due an progesterone insufficiency, such as luteal phase defect and a tendency to miscarriage, are mainly categorized as spleen-kidney dual vacuity patterns. Further, progesterone has recently proven to help prevent or slow down osteoporosis both in oral and transdermal form. In Chinese herbal medicine, it is kidney yang supplements mostly combined with liver blood and kidney yin supplements which are used to prevent bone degeneration.

The potential side effects of progesterone use (high blood pressure, heart disease, stroke, and high cholesterol levels) all tend to be related at least partially to either liver yang hyperactivity or a floating up of yang due to vacuity of yin. Such hyperactivity of liver yang or the creation of yin vacuity heat may, according to Chinese medical theory, be the side effects of over-supplementing yang qi in patients who do not have a yang qi vacuity.

Many Chinese herbal formulas used successfully for menopausal complaints are quite similar to formulas used for slightly younger women with infertility due to luteal phase defect and women with habitual miscarriages. Since it is known in Western medicine that luteal phase defect and habitual miscarriage are due to the corpus luteum is not secreting adequate amounts of progesterone, then Chinese herbal formulas effective both for preventing or easing menopausal symptoms and for correcting a luteal phase defect must be either supplementing a woman's progesterone or helping her body to produce it by some other mechanism.

Such Chinese herbs fall into two main categories: kidney yang supplements such as Herba Epimedii (*Xian Ling Pi*), Rhizoma Curculiginis Orchioidis (*Xian Mao*), Radix Morindae Officinalis (*Ba Ji Tian*), Radix Dipsaci (*Xu Duan*), and Cortex Eucommiae Ulmoidis (*Du Zhong*); and qi supplements such as Radix Panacis Ginseng (*Ren Shen*), Radix Astragali Membranacei (*Huang Qi*), and Rhizoma Atractylodis Macrocephalae (*Bai Zhu*). Dispsacus and Eucommia are not only commonly used to forestall a threatened miscarriage but are also commonly used to increase bone density in older patients. Therefore, we may infer that Chinese herbal medicinals used to treat menopausal and post-menopausal conditions such as bone loss, most definitely have the ability to supplement progesterone.

Other Western Therapies for Menopausal Complaints

While HRT is the most common therapy used for menopausal and postmenopausal women, there are other substances which are used in some situations. Androgens (male sex hormones) can be used for loss of sex drive and low energy. Thyroid hormones are sometimes used to good effect for women with low energy or wild energy swings. Diuretics are given for water retention and edema. Tranquilizers and sedatives are given for anxiety or sleep disturbances. All of these are helpful to some women, but all of them have possible side effects and all have the same drawback as was just described above. Because these Western medicines are not prescribed on the basis of an individualized pattern discrimination, Western doctors have no way of knowing who will react poorly to any given medicine other than by trial and error.

On the other hand, there are effective, noniatrogenic Chinese herbal remedies for *all* these accompanying signs and symptoms of menopause which work more gently and holistically to restore optimum balance to the body. When prescribed by a professionally trained practitioner, Chinese medicine has the know-how to determine just which herbs in what doses and combinations are right for which individual women. Thus there is healing without side effects. The only kind of true healing there is!

Summing Up

What we know is that HRT and other hormonal therapies commonly used for menopausal complaints are effective at reducing or eliminating many symptoms in the short term. We also know that they all have potential side effects and potentially serious risks with longterm use. In light of these unknowns, many women wish to find alternative therapies that have a safer track record. This book is designed to inform women that such alternatives exist and have been prescribed by Chinese doctors for 2,000 years.

OSTEOPOROSIS: ALTERNATIVE TREATMENT OPTIONS

Overview of Western Treatments

Osteoporosis (OP) is considered to be a major health problem in America today affecting as many as 20 million Americans, 90% of which are postmenopausal women. Approximately 50% of Caucasian women by the age of 75 will have spinal compression fractures.[45] The cost for treatment of osteoporosis in the U.S. is a staggering $7 billion annually and the disease is also associated with high mortality rates due to a variety of complications..

Primary OP is considered to have multiple causative factors including 1) failure to develop sufficient bone mass during youth, 2) excessive age related bone loss, 3) defective intestinal calcium absorption, 4) lowered blood estrogen levels beginning at menopause, and 5) sensitivity to parathyroid hormone calcitonin.[46]

For both preventive and remedial treatment of osteoporosis, Western medicine has many treatments. ERT is the primary one and has been considered to be quite effective in preventing osteoporosis, but must be continued for life for continued protection. This is whether or not other symptoms indicating ERT use are present. (See the previous chapter for information on ERT.) Other therapies include calcitonin, calcium carbonate supplementation, sodium

---

[45]   Gambrell Jr., Don. R., *op.cit.*, p. 65

[46]   Berkow, R., and Fletcher, A., *op.cit.*, p. 1296

fluoride, parathyroid hormone supplementation, and newer drugs called raloxifene, etidronate and alendronate. Patients are also encouraged to get regular exercise of a weight bearing nature.

Calcium Carbonate

This supplement is given in amounts of 2,400 to 3,600 milligrams per day. While it has the advantage of being very inexpensive, it is poorly absorbed by those with poor digestion because it causes an alkalinization of the stomach. Since hydrochloric acid (HCL) is necessary for the absorption of calcium in the intestine, an alkaline form of calcium is not really cost effective since it will not be as well absorbed, and it may cause further digestive difficulty by suppressing necessary HCL levels in the stomach. We will discuss other more effective sources of calcium below.

Calcitonin

Calcitonin is a peptide hormone secreted by the parathyroid gland which inhibits the rate of calcium coming out of the bones into the bloodstream. It is available from human, pork, and fish sources and is sometimes administered singly, or in conjunction with ERT or sodium fluoride. Side effects from calcitonin therapy may include nausea and vomiting, facial flushing, or local inflammatory reaction at the site of injection, as calcitonin is usually administered via injection.

Sodium Fluoride

Fluorine (fluoride) increases the deposition of calcium in the bones, thereby increasing their strength. It is often used in conjunction with ERT, calcitonin therapy, or calcium supplementation in the form of sodium fluoride. Although traces of this mineral are beneficial to the body, excessive amounts are definitely harmful, inhibiting various enzyme processes which are vital to the metabolism of vitamins, causing calcification of ligaments and tendons, and even degenerative changes in the kidneys, liver, central nervous system, and heart. Sodium fluoride is found in drinking water supplies throughout the U.S. today in order to prevent the decay of tooth enamel, although this form of fluorine is not the same as calcium fluoride which is how fluorine is found in nature. Sodium fluoride is toxic if it comprises more than two parts per million in water supplies. Women on long term sodium fluoride supplementation should have blood fluoride levels monitored regularly. It is interesting to note that calcium is a natural antidote to sodium fluoride poisoning. Seafoods, meat, cheeses, and certain types of tea are good sources of natural fluorine and, in general, fluorine deficiency is quite rare in the U.S.

Etidronate

Etidronate is a biphosphonate which works by inhibiting resorption of minerals by the blood from the bone. This is a new medicine for the treatment of osteoporosis and initial research studies with it are promising. Findings of a two year research study of 429 women with postmenopausal OP conducted by the Massachusetts Medical Society concluded that intermittent cyclic etidronate therapy for 12 months resulted in significant increases in bone mineral density which were sustained for another 12 months after discontinuing use of the drug.[47] The improvement in bone mass mostly affected the spine, while other areas such as wrist and hip bones did not respond positively to this drug. Few side effects to this drug appeared in this study. In another study done in 1991, Dr. Steven Harris noted several drawbacks to the use of etidronate and related drugs. In his

---

[47]   Watts, Nelson B., et al., "Intermittent Cyclic Etidronate Treatment of Postmenopausal Women with Osteoporosis", *The New England Journal of Medicine*, Vol. 323, #2, July 12, 1990, p. 73

study, three or more year users of these agents showed an actual increase in the incidence of hip fractures.[48]

Alendronate (Fosamax®)

Fosamax is a relatively new drug first synthesized by Merck Laboratories. This drug was tested on rats during NASA space flights, and has shown promise in helping prevent bone thinning.[49] It is a chemical relative of etidronate, described above, and can cause mild digestive system side effects.

Parathyroid hormone (PTH)

The use of this hormone seems to reverse some osteoporotic changes in women with the disease. Studies of this new therapy are promising in certain types of cases.[50]

Raloxifene

This is also a newer drug, marketed by Eli Lilly as Evista®, and is designed to fight osteoporosis by activating special estrogen receptors in bone. In early studies of this drug, it was shown to also reduce the risk of cancer by more than 50% and as much as 83% in

---

[48] Storm, T., Thamsborg, G., Steiniche, T., Genant H.K., Sorenson, O.H., "Effect of intermittent cyclical etidronate therapy on bone mass and fracture rate in women with postmenopausal osteoporosis," *New England Jrnl. of Med.*, 1900; 322: 1265-71.

[49] "Osteoporosis in Women", *Clinical Reference Systems*, December 1997, p. 2201

[50] "Osteoporosis: Studies Show Promise for Stronger Bones", Mike Briley, *Arthritis Today*, July-August, 1997, Vol. 1, #4, p. 10-11

post-menopausal women. Unlike its cousin, tamoxifen, it is not linked to increases in uterine cancer.[51]

New Research on ERT, Natural Progesterone, and Osteoporosis

While early studies on the effects of estrogen replacement for the treatment of osteoporosis appeared promising, more recent studies have questioned the benefits of estrogen for this use in light of the potential unacceptable side effects.[52] Even in authoritative medical textbooks such as the 18th edition (1988) of *Cecil's Textbook of Medicine*, the chapters on osteoporosis give only cautious statements regarding the use of estrogen, stating that "estrogen is more effective than calcium but has significant side effects."[53] In this context, it should be recalled that, above a certain minimum, calcium intake has no further effect on osteoporosis, so how much effect does estrogen replacement have?[54] In fact, when most studies in this field are looked at more closely, true gains in bone mass or

---

[51]   "Tracking a Cancer Cure: A Sheaf of New Studies Shed More Light on Ways to Combat a Killer," *US News & World Report*, June 1, 1998, Vol. 124, #21, P. 52

[52]   Barbel, U.S., "Estrogens in the prevention and treatment of post-menopausal osteoporosis; a review", *Amer. Jour. of Med.*, 1988; 85:847-850.

[53]   *Cecil's Textbook of Medicine*, 18th Edition, 1988, p. 1514.

[54]   Riis, B.R., Thomsen, K, Christiansen, C., "Does calcium supplementation prevent postmenopausal bone loss?", *N. Engl. J. of Med.*, 1987; 316: 173-177.

reductions in urinary calcium excretion were found only when progesterone was part of the hormone replacement.[55]

While it appears that estrogen definitely plays a role in preventing bone resorption by the blood, it has little or no effect at all on new bone formation. Progesterone, on the other hand, has shown positive effects on bone formation in many studies.[56] One doctor has reported using transdermal progesterone, *i.e.*, progesterone cream, on his patients, regardless of estrogen use. With regular bone mineral density (BMD) tests using photo absorptiometry, his patients experienced increases of up to 15% in BMD in six months, and up to 25% in three years. The median three year increase was 15%. These benefits were independent of age, time from menopause, or estrogen use.[57] In the discussion of Chinese herbal medicine and ERT in

[55] Christiansen C., Christen M.S., Transbol I., "Bone mass in postmenopausal women after withdrawal of oestrogen/gastragen replacement therapy." *Lancet*, 1981, Feb. 28; 459-461

Lindsay R., Hart, D.M., Purdie D., Ferguson M.M., Clark, A.S., Kraszewski, A., "Comparative effects of oestrogen and a progestogen on bone loss in postmenopausal women." *Clin. Sc. & Mol. Medicine*, 1978; 54-193-195.

Christiansen, C., Riis B.J., Nilas L., Rodbro P., Deftos L., "Uncoupling of bone formation and resorption by combined oestrogen and progestogen therapy in postmenopausal osteoporosis. *Lancet*, 1985, Oct. 12: 800-801.

[56] Prior, J.C., Vigna, Y.M., "Spinal bone loss and ovulatory disturbances," *New Eng. J. of Med., 1990*; 323:1221-7.

Prior, J.C., Vigna, Y.M.,, Alojado, N., "Progesterone and the prevention of osteoporosis." *Canadian Journal of OB Gyn & Women's Health Care*, 1991; 3:178-184.

Lee, J.R., "Osteoporosis reversal; the role of progesterone," *Intern'l. Clinical Nutrition Review*, 1990; 10:384-391.

[57] Lee, J.R., "Is Natural Progesterone the missing link in osteoporosis prevention and treatment?" *Medical Hypotheses*, 1991; 35:316-318.

previous chapter, I have suggested definite Chinese medical corroboration for these studies.

Based upon these reports, it seems that while estrogen may have a small impact on osteoporosis, progesterone, even when administered in its safer, transdermal form, is a more powerful tool for preventing or reversing osteoporosis. Clinical reports seem to bear this out. However, it is more important yet to remember that similar effects may be accomplished by using Chinese medicinals without using Western hormone replacement and, therefore, avoiding the potential side effects of these substances. For anyone interested in seeing further research on the subject of natural progesterone there is a book, *Natural Progesterone: The Multiple Roles of a Remarkable Hormone*, listed in the Suggested Reading section of this book.

Alternative Therapies

While Western medicine has a number of therapeutic options for OP, it continues to be a major problem in postmenopausal women in the U.S. as the statistics above indicate. In light of this, effective prevention and alternative therapies for this problem, especially ones which can be used safely over an extended period of time, would be a welcome addition.

Microcrystalline Hydroxyapatite (MCHC)

The most promising new, natural, vitamin/mineral supplement for the treatment and prevention of osteoporosis is microcrystalline hydroxyapatite (MCHC). This is a whole bone extract that has been shown to improve calcium absorption. MCHC does not have the drawbacks of most calcium preparations because it is a compound containing the bone minerals calcium, phosphorus, magnesium, and fluoride in the normal physiological proportions. Not only has this substance been found to halt bone loss, but actually to restore bone mass in cases of OP.[58] It can be used both remedially and preventively, without side effects.

Metagenics, Inc. has two MCHC formulas. Cal-Apatite™ is an MCHC formula for people who are already taking a multivitamin/mineral supplement. Osteogenics™ is a more complete mineral formula designed for those who are not taking adequate minerals from any other source. Other companies may have similar formulas, and it is probably wise to consult a health practitioner before beginning any long term supplementation program.

Traditionally in Chinese medicine, doctors prescribed various types of animal bones for the treatment of joint and low back pain in older patients. The most famous of these, tiger bone (Os Tigridis, *Hu Gu*), is a main cause for the threatened extinction of this beautiful species. Happily, Chinese doctors no longer have to prescribe tiger bone. Western research suggests that any form of whole bone extract is effective for the purpose of building bones, and although there are many Chinese patent medicine still on the market which advertise that they contain tiger bone, these should never be used. This is one place where Western scientific research has most assuredly improved upon the wisdom of Chinese medicine.

Herbal Remedies

As was stated earlier in this book, according to Chinese medicine, the bones are ruled by the kidneys, while the sinews are ruled by the liver. The sinews and the bones are always spoken of together as a unit in Chinese medicine. Since aging largely involves the degeneration of the kidneys, problems with bone loss, bone softening, arthritis, etc. associated with aging are not surprising.

---

[58]   Dixon, Allan St. J., "Non-hormonal Treatment of Osteoporosis", *British Medical Journal*, Vol 286, #6370, March, 1983, p. 999

The Chinese have largely treated aging problems of the bones, therefore, by supplementing kidney yang and nourishing liver blood.

There are a number of effective herbal formulas for doing this, with many research studies supporting their effectiveness for prevention and treatment of bones loss. These formulas typically include the same medicinals discussed in the previous chapter under progesterone. They include Cortex Eucommiae Ulmoidis (*Du Zhong*), Radix Dipsaci (*Xu Duan*), Radix Morindae Officinalis (*Ba Ji Tian*), Rhizoma Curculiginis Orchioidis (*Xian Mao*), and Herba Epimedii (*Xian Ling Pi*). When these kinds of Chinese medicinals are combined with whole bone extract sources of calcium and are properly prescribed on the basis of a professional Chinese medical pattern discrimination, they can be take over a long period of time without side

Other Preventive Measures

It is well known that regular weight-bearing exercise is crucial to the maintenance of bone mass. It is also important to know what activities or substances will deplete bone mass or speed up its loss. The list is not surprising, although some of us will be surprised/disappointed to know about all the things which we should avoid.

1. Excessive alcohol causes malabsorption of many vitamins and minerals including zinc, which is required for the synthesis of vitamin D_3, which is in turn required for bone mineralization.

2. Antacid products which contain aluminum (many over the counter products do). These increase the urinary and fecal excretion of calcium. Cooking with aluminum pots and pans has a similar effect. For people with hyperacidic digestive discomfort, there are other natural products on the market which will not cause this

problem or other problems which may be related to aluminum ingestion.

3. Soft drinks, especially those with caffeine, cause significant increase in urinary calcium loss.[59]

4. Prolonged or repeated use of antibiotics, especially broad spectrum types, may directly affect calcium balance in the body. In a study by Lois Kramer and colleagues, it was noted that tetracycline use for three months induced significant increase in urinary calcium output and adversely affected collagen synthesis as well.[60]

5. Smoking accelerates bone loss as shown in studies comparing vertebral fracture levels in smokers and nonsmokers.[61]

6. Caffeine. See #3 above. Everyone should know that caffeine is a drug, not a food. For an overview, see chapter eight on diet, page 110 of this book. A plethora of studies in recent years have attested to the relationship between caffeine consumption and osteoporosis.

7. Excess phytic acid found in many unprocessed grains prevents the absorption of calcium into the bone. Grains which are partially processed, i.e., part of the bran is removed, are lower in phytic acid. This is interesting in light of the fact that in Chinese dietary theory, all grains should be at least partially processed for easier digestion.

---

[59] Hollingberry, P.W., and Massey, L.K., "Effect of Dietary Caffeine and Sucrose on Urinary Calcium Excretion in Adolescents", Fed. Proc., #45, Abstract, 1986, p. 1286

[60] Kramer, Lois, et al., "Drug-Mineral Interactions", Fed. Proc., Vol. 43, #4, Abstract, 1281, 1986, p. 375

[61] Daniell, H.W., "Osteoporosis of the Slender Smoker: Vertebral Compression Fractures & Loss of Metacarpal Cortex in Relation to Postmenopausal Cigarette Smoking & Lack of Obesity", Arch. Internal Medicine, #136, 1976, p. 398-404

People who eat large amounts of bran should take higher amounts of calcium.

This list is not exhaustive. There are many other Western drugs and procedures which may affect bone mineralization including corticosteroids, Dilantin, oral contraceptives, isoniazid, nystatin, hemodialysis, and gastric surgery.

Additionally, people with lactose intolerance, hyperthyroidism, or diabetes, are known to absorb minerals poorly or have insufficient amounts in their diet. Such people should supplement their diets with multi-mineral products, preferably those which contain MCHC compounds.

Summing Up

Although osteoporosis and bone demineralization has undoubtedly been a problem for human beings for centuries, it is also probable that a sedentary lifestyle plus the increased consumption of caffeine, sugar, antibiotics, steroid drugs, aluminum-containing antacids, nicotine, and soft drinks seen in late 20th century America exacerbates the problem. Along with preventive measures related to the above, people with high risk levels for OP would be well advised to supplement their diets with easily absorbable minerals, especially calcium.

Ninety per cent of the people who experience OP in the U.S. are postmenopausal women. Although Western drug intervention, especially ERT, has some effect for preventing and treating OP, studies suggest that it is possible to treat and prevent it effectively through more natural methods which do not involve the possible risks of hormone therapy along with regular weight bearing exercise.

While the jury is still out on which methods are most effective with the fewest side effects, there are many women who cannot or do not wish to do ERT. For these women, Chinese herbal medicine offers a very real, very welcome alternative. A description of a recent Chinese study on the effects of Chinese herbs on senile osteoporosis (*i.e.*, osteoporosis in older people) is given in the next chapter.

CHINESE MEDICAL RESEARCH ON MENOPAUSAL SYNDROME

Considerable research has been done in the People's Republic of China on the effects of acupuncture and Chinese herbal medicine on all aspects of menopausal syndrome. Usually, this research is in the form of a clinical audit. That means that a group of patients with the same diseases, patterns, or major complaints are given the same treatment for a certain period of time. After this time, the patients are counted to see how many were cured, how many got a marked effect, how many got some effect, and how many got no effect. This kind of "outcome-based research" has, up until only very recently, not been considered credible in the West where, for the last 30 years or so, the double-blind, placebo-controlled comparison study has been considered the "gold standard." However, such double-blind, placebo-controlled comparison studies are impossible to design in Chinese medicine and do not, in any case, measure effectiveness in a real-life situation.

Clinical audits, on the other hand, do measure actual clinical satisfaction in real-life patients. Such clinical audits may not exclude the patient's trust and belief in the therapist or the therapy as an important component in the result. However, real-life is not as neat and discreet as a controlled laboratory experiment. If the majority of patients are satisfied with the results of a particular treatment and there are no adverse side effects to that treatment, then that is good enough for the Chinese doctor, and, in my experience, that is also good enough for the vast majority of my patients.

Below are abbreviated translations of several recent research articles published in Chinese medical journals on the treatment of menopausal syndrome and one on osteoporosis. I think that most women with menopausal complaints and issues reading these statistics would think that Chinese medicine was worth a try. I do.

"The Treatment of 22 Cases of Menopausal Syndrome" by Cao Guo-rong, *Guo Yi Lun Tan (Forum on Chinese Medicine)*, Vol. 11, #5, 1996, p. 37

In the last few years, the author applied *Bu Xin Tang Jia Wei* (Supplement the Heart Decoction with Added Flavors) for treating 22 cases of menopausal syndrome. Among the 22 cases, 14 cases were between the ages of 44-49; while eight cases were between 49-53. The duration of illness was, in 15 cases, from 6 months to one year. In the other six cases, it was from 1-2 years.

Treatment method

Every case in this group was treated with *Bu Xin Tang Jia Wei*. The ingredients were: cooked Radix Rehmanniae (*Shu Di*), uncooked Radix Rehmanniae (*Sheng Di*), Radix Scrophulariae Ningpoensis (*Xuan Shen*), Semen Ziziphi Spinosae (*Suan Zao Ren*), Tuber Ophiopogonis Japonici (*Mai Dong*), Tuber Asparagi Cochinensis (*Tian Dong*), Radix Salviae Miltiorrhizae (*Dan Shen*), Sclerotium Poriae Cocos (*Fu Ling*), Radix Angelicae Sinensis (*Dang Gui*), 12g @; Fructus Schisandrae Chinensis (*Wu Wei Zi*), Radix Codonopsitis Pilosulae (*Dang Shen*), Semen Biotae Orientalis (*Bai Zi Ren*), Radix Polygalae Tenuifoliae (*Yuan Zhi*), Cortex Radicis Lycii Chinensis (*Di Gu Pi*), 10g @; Concha Ostreae (*Mu Li*), Os Draconis (*Long Gu*), 20g @; Radix Platycodi Grandiflori (*Jie Geng*), 6g; and Cinnabaris (*Zhu Sha*), 2g. Every day, one *ji* was decocted in water [and administered]. The additions and subtractions were as follows: If there was head pain and dizziness, Rhizoma Gastrodiae Elatae

(*Tian Ma*) and Ramulus Uncariae Cum Uncis (*Gou Teng*) were added to nourish the liver. If there was ear ringing, Magnetitum (*Ci Shi*) was added to suppress yang. If there was skin itching, Periostracum Cicadae (*Chan Tui*) and Fructus Tribuli Terrestris (*Bai Ji Li*) were added to dispel wind.

Treatment results

After taking these medicinals, this group obtained full recovery, and all symptoms disappeared. The number of *ji* or packets of herbs administered ranged from 8-32; and all cases without exception got a good response.

Case history

Female, age 49, cadre; initial visit was on March 2, 1992. During the last year, this patient's menstrual cycle had gradually lengthened and the amount of her menses had lessened. There was heart vexation, easy anger, insomnia, and heart palpitations. Her head and face regions suddenly got hot and there was sweating, heat in the palms and soles, and sometimes dry, bound stools. The tongue fur was thin and white; the tongue body was pale red. The pulse was fine and rapid. The pattern was kidney yin insufficiency with vacuous yang floating astray and heart blood insufficiency with the heart not being nourished. The treatment principles were to enrich yin and subdue yang, nourish the heart and calm the spirit. The treatment used was *Bu Xin Tang Jia Wei*. After administering four *ji* of these medicinals, all the patient's symptoms were alleviated. After continuing with four more *ji*, all the symptoms were entirely eliminated.

Author's Discussion

Chinese medicine refers to menopausal syndrome as "before and after the severance of the menses various symptoms." Women bear

173

children, have periods, and, in later years, go through the transitional stage of menopause. The main reasons for menopause are the kidney qi gradually becoming vacuous and the gradual exhaustion of the *tian gui*. In addition, the two channels, the *chong* and *ren*, become debilitated and scanty. When this happens, a series of symptoms emerges. Yin vacuity with yang hyperactivity and heart blood insufficiency are the major patterns. Therefore, the treatment principles are to enrich yin and subdue yang, nourish the heart and calm the spirit. This prescription centers on cooked Rehmannia to enrich yin and supplement the kidneys, while uncooked Rehmannia, Ophiopogon, and Asparagus enrich yin and clear heat. Scrophularia is used to invigorate water and restrain fire. Dang Gui and Salvia are used to supplement the blood and nourish the heart. Cinnabar enters the heart channel and settles the heart. Ziziphus and Biota are used to nourish the heart and calm the spirit. Poria boosts the heart qi. Polygala promotes the interaction of the heart and kidneys. Schisandra engenders fluids and constrains sweat. Cortex Lycii abates vacuity heat. Oyster Shell and Dragon Bone subdue yang, secure and astringe. Platycodon carries the medicinals upward. When all these medicinals are combined, together they have the effect of enriching yin and subduing yang, nourishing the heart and calming the spirit. Since the prescription suits the symptoms, the results were satisfactory.

"Supplement Kidneys & Quiet the Heart Method to Treat Menopause: A Summary of 58 Cases" by Guo Xiao-ming, *Yun Nan Zhong Yi Zhong Yao Za Zhi (Yunnan Journal of Chinese Medicine & Materia Medica)*, #5, 1996, p. 19

The author, on the basis of Chinese medical theory, used the treatment methods of supplementing the kidneys and quieting the heart to obtain the results related below. Altogether there were 58 women. Eight were between the ages of 41-45, 36 were between 46-50, 12 were 51-55, and two were 56 years of age or older. The shortest duration of illness was one month; the longest was 10 years. Menstrual circumstances: Natural menopause, 11 cases. Those still menstruating but having chaotic or irregular menses, 47 cases.

The major symptoms were dizziness, ear ringing, heart palpitations, disquieted heart, agitation, easy anger, tidal heat, sweating, vexatious heat in the five hearts (*i.e.*, the palms of the hands, soles of the feet, and heart region of the chest), insomnia, and dream-disturbed sleep. Irregularity of the menses was the essential diagnostic criterion. Among these women, two distinct patterns were discriminated:

1. Predominant yin vacuity pattern (43 cases or 74.2%)
The symptoms were tidal heat (*i.e.* hot flashes), sweating, vexatious heat in the five hearts, insomnia, and dream-disturbed sleep, heart vexation, easy anger, dizziness, ear ringing or skin itching, dry mouth, bound stools, yellow, scanty urine, irregular menstrual periods, and bright red colored menses. The tongue tip was red, and the pulse was fine and rapid.

2. Predominant yang vacuity pattern (15 cases or 25.8%)
The symptoms were tidal heat, sweating, heart vexation, easy anger, heart palpitations, disquieted heart, insomnia, dream-disturbed sleep, dizziness, ear ringing, depression, anxiety, painful aching lumbus, fatigued spirit and lack of strength, cold body and limbs, sloppy, thin stools, frequent urination, or menses pale in color. The tongue was pale red and predominantly fat with white fur. The pulse was deep and fine.

175

Treatment method

The basic formula was composed of: cooked Radix Rehmannia (*Shu Di*), Fructus Corni Officinalis (*Zao Pi*), Fructus Lycii Chinensis (*Gou Qi Zi*), calcined Os Draconis (*Long Gu*), calcined Concha Ostreae (*Mu Li*), and the crowns of Nelumbo Nucifera (*He Ding*). Then, according to the pattern discrimination, additions and subtractions were made.

For the predominant yin vacuity pattern: stir-fried Semen Ziziphi Spinosae (*Zao Ren*), Fructus Schisandrae Chinensis (*Wu Wei Zi*), Fructus Ligustri Lucidi (*Nu Zhen Zi*), Tuber Ophiopogonis Japonici (*Mai Dong*), and Herba Dendrobii (*Shi Hu*) were added. If there was skin itching or the feeling of insects moving on the skin, Cortex Radicis Moutan (*Dan Pi*) and Fructus Tribuli Terrestris (*Bai Ji Li*) were added to clear heat, cool the blood, and dispel wind. If the mouth was dry and the stools were bound, Radix Scrophulariae Ningpoensis (*Xuan Shen*) and processed Radix Polygoni Multiflori (*Shou Wu*) were added. If the menstrual period was chaotic [*i.e.*, irregular] or the menses were bright red and incessantly dripping, Gelatinum Corii Asini (*E Jiao*), Radix Scrophulariae Ningpoensis (*Xuan Shen*), and Herba Agrimoniae Pilosae (*Xian He Cao*) were added to supplement and cool the blood and stop bleeding.

For the predominant yang vacuity pattern: Cortex Eucommiae Ulmoidis (*Du Zhong*), Semen Cuscutae Chinensis (*Tu Si Zi*), and Radix Achyranthis Bidentatae (*Niu Xi*) were added. If the stools were sloppy and urination was frequent, then Cortex Cinnamomi Cassiae (*Rou Gui*) and Fructus Psoraleae Corylifoliae (*Bu Gu Zhi*) were added to warm the kidneys, reinforce yang, and stop diarrhea. If the color of the menses was pale and there was cold pain in the lower back, Cortex Cinnamomi Cassiae (*Rou Gui*), Radix Angelicae Sinensis (*Dang Gui*), and Folium Artemisiae Argyii (*Ai Ye*) were added to warm the uterus and supplement the blood.

176

Curative criteria & results

After undergoing treatment with 6-8 *ji* of these medicinals, if the main symptoms disappeared and the accompanying symptoms improved or lessened, this was considered improvement. If the main symptoms or accompanying symptoms clearly improved or ameliorated, this was considered a change for the better. Unchanged symptoms were considered no result. During the time of taking the formula, other medicinal teas were stopped. After treatment, this group had 48 cases with marked improvement and 10 cases changed for the better.

"A Clinical Analysis of 557 Cases of Menopausal Syndrome" by Zhang Da-ying, *Tian Jin Zhong Yi (Tianjin Chinese Medicine)*, #3, 1994, p. 7-8

Since 1960, the author has treated 557 cases of menopausal syndrome based on a discrimination of patterns with very good results. Typically, the onset of this condition occurs between 45-55 years of age with an average age of 48. If the menstruation ceases in the early 40s and the symptoms of this syndrome appear, this is called premature menopause. If, on the other hand, menstruation does not cease until 55, this is referred to as late onset menopause. Of the 557 cases in this study, the onset of this condition occurred between 45-54 years of age in 292 cases or 78.4%. Premature menopause occurred in 62 cases or 11.9%. Late onset menopause occurred in 51 cases or 9.7%.

In 517 cases or 89.2%, menstruation had become irregular before ceasing. In 510 cases or 90%, there was insomnia. In 488 cases or 87.6%, there was difficulty falling asleep, sleep which was not deep, excessive dreams, tenseness, agitation and easy anger, and restlessness when sitting or lying down. Four hundred twenty-five cases or 76.3% had tidal heat (*i.e.*, hot flashes) and sweating. Other symptoms included chest oppression, a suffocated feeling, a tense feeling in the precordial region, diminished appetite, loose stools, abnormal blood pressure, nonspecific aches and pains, abnormal sexual desire, swelling and distention in the body and limbs, tinnitus, etc.

1. Yin vacuity, yang hyperactivity pattern: 226 cases or 47.8%

Main symptoms: Tidal heat, sweating, insomnia, excessive dreams, dizziness, tinnitus, low back, leg, and foot pain, poor memory, vexation and agitation, a red tongue with scant coating, and a wiry, fine, rapid pulse

Treatment principles: Enrich yin and subdue yang, settle, still, and quiet the spirit

Formula: *Geng Nian An Tang* (Climacteric Quieting Decoction)

Ingredients: Uncooked and cooked Radix Rehmanniae (*Sheng Shu Di*), 30g @, Radix Polygoni Multiflori (*He Shou Wu*), 15g, Rhizoma Alismatis (*Ze Xie*), 10g, Sclerotium Poriae Cocos (*Fu Ling*), 15g, Cortex Radicis Moutan (*Dan Pi*), 10g, Radix Scrophulariae Ningpoensis (*Xuan Shen*), 15g, Tuber Ophiopogonis Japonici (*Mai Dong*), 15g, Fructus Schisandrae Chinensis (*Wu Wei Zi*), 10g, Fructus Corni Officinalis (*Shan Zhu Yu*), 10g

If sweating was excessive, Fructus Levis Tritici (*Fu Xiao Mai*) and aged Semen Setariae Italicae (*Kang Gu Lao*) were added. If there was heart vexation, Fructus Gardeniae Jasminoidis (*Zhi Zi*) and Semen Praeparatus Sojae (*Dan Dou Chi*) were added. If there was excessive dreams, Hangzhou Radix Albus Paeoniae Lactiflorae

178

(*Hang Shao*), Fructus Chaenomelis Lagenariae (*Mu Gua*) were added. If there was insomnia, Magnetitum (*Ci Shi*), Concha Margaritiferae (*Zhen Zhu Mu*), and Caulis Polygoni Multiflori (*Ye Jiao Teng*) were added. If there was headache, Fructus Viticis (*Man Jing Zi*), Radix Angelicae Dahuricae (*Bai Zhi*), and Flos Chrysanthemi Morifolii (*Ju Hua*) were added. If there was dizziness, Herba Dendrobii (*Shi Hu*), Radix Platycodi Grandiflori (*Jie Geng*), and Radix Glycyrrhizae (*Gan Cao*) were added. And if there was low back and leg pain, Radix Dipsaci (*Chuan Duan*), Ramulus Loranthi Seu Visci (*Ji Sheng*), and Radix Achyranthis Bidentatae (*Niu Xi*) were added.

Chinese patent medicines: *Geng Nian An* (Quieting the Climacteric), *i.e.*, the above formula made into tablet form; *Wu Wei Zi Chong Ji* (Schisandra Soluble Granules); *Liu Wei Di Huang Wan* (Six Flavors Rehmannia Pills); *Er Zhi Wan* (Two Ultimates Pills); *Da Bu Yin Wan* (Great Supplementing Yin Pills); and *Zuo Gui Wan* (Restore the Left [Kidney] Pills) can also be administered.

Acupuncture/moxibustion: Points chosen included *Tai Xi* (Ki 3), *San Yin Jiao* (Sp 6), *Tai Chong* (Liv 3), *Shui Gou* (GV 26), and *Nei Guan* (Per 6). If there was headache, *Lie Que* (Lu 7) was added. If there was dizziness, *Yin Tang* (M-HN-3) was added. If there was excessive sweating, *He Gu* (LI 4) and *Fu Liu* (Ki 7) were added.

2. Qi stagnation, blood stasis pattern: 256 cases or 46%

Main symptoms: Heart vexation, easy anger, rib-side distention and pain or piercing pain in the periphery of the body, vexatious heat within the heart, tidal heat, sweating, heart palpitations, insomnia, a bowstring or choppy pulse, and a bluish purple tongue or static spots and patches on the tongue

179

Treatment principles: Quicken the blood and transform stasis, eliminate vexation and quiet the spirit

Formula: *Xue Fu Zhu Yu Tang* (Dispel Stasis from the Blood Mansion Decoction)

If there was insomnia, Succinum (*Hu Bo*) and Caulis Polygoni Multiflori (*Ye Jiao Teng*) were added. If there was heart vexation, Fructus Gardeniae Jasminoidis (*Zhi Zi*) and Semen Praeparatus Sojae (*Dan Dou Chi*) were added. If there were heart palpitations, Radix Salviae Miltiorrhizae (*Dan Shen*) and Radix Polygalae Tenuifoliae (*Yuan Zhi*) were added.

Chinese patent medicines: *Fu Fang Dan Shen Pian* (Compound Salvia Tablets); *Xue Fu Zhu Yu Jiao Nong* (Dispel Stasis from the Blood Mansion Gelatin Capsules)

Acupuncture/moxibustion: *Xue Hai* (Sp 10), *San Yin Jiao* (Sp 6), *Tian Shu* (St 25), *Zhang Men* (Liv 13)

3. Phlegm dampness internally obstructing pattern: 35 cases or 6.8%

Main symptoms: Dizziness, muffled feeling head, vacuity edema of the facial region, bodily swelling or floating edema of the face and limbs, sweating, tidal heat, torpid intake (*i.e.*, poor appetite), chest oppression, loose stools, vacuity vexation, insomnia, a fat tongue with a thick, slimy or damp, glossy coating, and a slightly slow or slippery pulse

Treatment principles: Dispel dampness and transform phlegm, fortify the spleen and harmonize the stomach

180

Formula: *Wen Dan Tang Jia Wei* (Warm the Gallbladder Decoction with Added Flavors)

If there was abdominal distention, Pericarpium Arecae Catechu (*Da Fu Pi*), 10g, and Semen Raphani Sativi (*Lai Fu Zi*), 10g, were added. If there was indigestion, Massa Medica Fermentatae (*Liu Qu*) and Corneum Endothelium Gigeriae Galli (*Nei Jin*) were added. If there was phlegm misting the portals of the heart, Rhizoma Arisaematis (*Nan Xing*), 10g, and Rhizoma Acori Graminei (*Chang Pu*), 10g, were added.

Chinese patent medicines: *Ju Hong Hua Tan Wan* (Red Citrus Peel Transform Phlegm Pills) and fresh bamboo juice (*Xian Zhu Li*) can also be used.

Acupuncture/moxibustion: *Feng Long* (St 40), *Di Ji* (Sp 8), *San Li* (St 36), *Li Gou* (Liv 5), *Shui Gou* (GV 26)

Of the 557 patients treated with the above protocols, 18 cases or 3.2% were completely cured, 227 cases or 40.8% were markedly improved, 298 cases or 53.5% got some results, and 14 cases or 2.5% got no result. Thus the total amelioration rate was 97.5%. It should be noted that some of the patients also received some tranquilizers, such as Valium, for short periods (1-2 weeks) and psychotherapy.

"Experiences in the Treatment of 52 Cases of Senile Osteoporosis with *Qing E Wan Jia Wei* (Young Pretty Girl Pills with Added Flavors)" by Shen Lin *et al., Hu Bei Zhong Yi Za Zhi (Hubei Journal of Chinese Medicine)*, #3, 1994, p. 16-18

Of the 52 patients treated in this clinical audit, 14 were men and 38 were women. They ranged in age from a young of 52 to an old of 78 years with an average age of 64.2 years old. All were seen as out-patients and all had some degree of upper and lower back pain. All the patients also were categorized as pertaining to various kidney vacuity patterns. There were 29 cases of kidney vacuity pattern, 12 cases of kidney yin vacuity pattern, 4 cases of kidney yang vacuity pattern, and 7 cases of kidney yin and yang dual vacuity pattern.

Qing E Wan Jia Wei consisted of: Cortex Eucommiae Ulmoidis (*Du Zhong*), Semen Juglandis Regiae (*Hu Tao Rou*), Fructus Psoraleae Corylifoliae (*Bu Gu Zhi*), Herba Epimedii (*Yin Yang Huo*), dry Radix Rehmanniae (*Gan Di Huang*), Radix Achyranthis Bidentatae (*Huai Niu Xi*), 12g @. These were decocted down into a pure, thick liquid. This was then sterilized under high pressure and bottled. Each day, these patients took this liquid orally, 20ml per time, 2 times per day, for 3 months. During this time they were prohibited to take other Chinese or Western medicinals.

After 15 days of taking these medicinals, 15 patients or 28.85% felt that their lower and upper back aching and pain was decreased. After 1 month, 37 cases or 71.15% felt their back pain decreased. After 2 months, 45 cases or 86.53% felt their back pain decreased. And after taking these medicinals for 3 months, 46 cases or 88.46% felt their back pain eliminated or decreased. Measurement s of bone density and x-ray analysis also showed statistically significant improvements from before to after this treatment.

182

The author cites the TCM statement of belief that the kidneys rule the bones as the rational for this treatment's design and efficacy. *Qing E Wan* is an ancient formula for supplementing the kidneys and that is why it is capable of treating this disease with good results. It is comprised of Eucommia, Psoralea, and Walnuts. It is capable of treating kidney qi vacuity weakness and strengthening the sinews and bones. In addition, Epimedium boosts the essence qi and supplements the low back and knees, while Rehmannia nourishes yin blood and fulfills the bone marrow. And Achyranthes leads the qi and blood to move downward, thus eliminating low back and knee bone pain. This formula is appropriate for the treatment of senile osteoporosis whether due to kidney vacuity, kidney yin vacuity, kidney yang vacuity, or kidney yin and yang dual vacuity.

FINDING A PROFESSIONAL PRACTITIONER OF CHINESE MEDICINE

Traditional Chinese medicine is one of the fastest growing holistic health care systems in the West today. At the present time, there are 50 colleges in the United States alone which offer 3-4 year training programs in acupuncture, moxibustion, Chinese herbal medicine, and Chinese medical massage. In addition, many of the graduates of these programs have done postgraduate studies at colleges and hospitals in China, Taiwan, Hong Kong, and Japan. Further, a growing number of trained Oriental medical practitioners have immigrated from China, Japan, and Korea to practice acupuncture and Chinese herbal medicine in the West.

Traditional Chinese medicine, including acupuncture, is a discreet and independent health care profession. It is not simply a technique that can easily be added to the array of techniques of some other health care profession. The study of Chinese medicine, acupuncture, and Chinese herbs is as rigorous as is the study of allopathic, chiropractic, naturopathic, or homeopathic medicine. Previous training in any one of these other systems does not automatically confer competence or knowledge in Chinese medicine. In order to get the full benefits and safety of Chinese medicine, one should seek out professionally trained and credentialed practitioners.

In the United States, recognition that acupuncture and Chinese medicine are their own independent professions has led to the creation of the National Commission for the Certification of Acupuncture & Oriental Medicine (NCCAOM). This commission has created and administers a national board examination in both acupuncture and Chinese herbal medicine in order to insure minimum levels of professional competence and safety. Those who pass the acupuncture exam append the letters Dipl. Ac. (Diplomate of Acupuncture) after their names, while those who pass the Chinese herbal exam use the letters Dipl. C.H. (Diplomate of Chinese Herbs). I recommend that persons wishing to experience the benefits of acupuncture and Chinese medicine should seek treatment in the U.S. only from those who are NCCAOM certified.

In addition, in the United States, acupuncture is a legal, independent health care profession in more than half the states. A few other states require acupuncturists to work under the supervision of M.D.s, while in a number of states, acupuncture has yet to receive legal status. In states where acupuncture is licensed and regulated, the names of acupuncture practitioners can be found in the *Yellow Pages* of your local phone book or through contacting your State Department of Health, Board of Medical Examiners, or Department of Regulatory Agencies. In states without licensure, it is doubly important to seek treatment only from NCCAOM diplomates.

When seeking a qualified and knowledgeable practitioner, word of mouth referrals are important. Satisfied patients are the most reliable credential a practitioner can have. It is appropriate to ask the practitioner for references from previous patients treated for the same problem. It is best to work with a practitioner who communicates effectively enough for the patient to feel understood and for the Chinese medical diagnosis and treatment plan to make sense. In all cases, a professional practitioner of Chinese medicine should be able and willing to give a written traditional Chinese diagnosis of the patient's pattern upon request.

For further information regarding the practice of Chinese medicine and acupuncture in the United States of America and for referrals to local professional associations and practitioners in the United States, prospective patients may contact:

National Commission for the Certification of Acupuncture & Oriental Medicine
11 Canal Center Plaza
Suite 300
Alexandria, VA 22314
Tel: (703) 548-9004
Fax: (202) 548-9079

The National Acupuncture & Oriental Medicine Alliance
14637 Starr Rd, SE
Olalla, WA 98357
Tel: (206) 851-6895
Fax: (206) 728-4841
email: 76143.2061@compuserve.com

The American Association of Oriental Medicine
433 Front St.
Catasauqua, PA 18032-2506
Tel: (610) 433-2448
Fax: (610) 433-1832

Learning More About Chinese Medicine

For more information on Chinese medicine in general, see:

The Web That Has No Weaver: Understanding Chinese Medicine by Ted Kaptchuk, Congdon & Weed, NY, 1983. This is the best overall introduction to Chinese medicine for the serious lay reader. It has been a standard since it was first published over a dozen years ago and it has yet to be replaced.

Chinese Secrets of Health & Longevity by Bob Flaws, Sound True, Boulder, CO, 1996. This is a six tape audiocassette course introducing Chinese medicine to laypeople. It covers basic Chinese medical theory, Chinese dietary therapy, Chinese herbal medicine, acupuncture, *qi gong, feng shui,* deep relaxation, life-style, and more.

Fundamentals of Chinese Medicine by the East Asian Medical Studies Society, Paradigm Publications, Brookline, MA, 1985. This is a more technical introduction and overview of Chinese medicine intended for professional entry level students.

Traditional Medicine in Contemporary China by Nathan Sivin, Center for Chinese Studies, University of Michigan, Ann Arbor, 1987. This book discusses the development of Chinese medicine in China in the last half century.

Imperial Secrets of Health and Longevity by Bob Flaws, Blue Poppy Press, Inc. Boulder, CO, 1994. This book includes a section on Chinese dietary therapy and generally introduces the basic concepts of good health according to Chinese medicine.

The Mystery of Longevity by Liu Zheng-cai, Foreign Languages Press, Beijing, 1990. This book is also about general principles and practices promoting good health according to Chinese medicine.

For more information on Chinese gynecology, see:

A Handbook of Chinese Menstrual Diseases by Bob Flaws, Blue Poppy Press, Boulder, CO, 1997. This book is meant as a professional text on the diagnosis and treatment of menstrual disease according to Chinese medicine. Within Chinese gynecology, menopausal syndrome is considered a menstrual disease. It also contains excellent chapters on basic Chinese gynecological theory and an especially good section on PMS. This book has set the professional standard in the Western practice of Chinese gynecology.

A Handbook of Traditional Chinese Gynecology by the Zhejiang College of TCM, translated by Zhang Ting-liang & Bob Flaws, Blue Poppy Press, Boulder, CO, 1995. This book is a translation of a standard Chinese gynecology meant for entry-level professional students in the People's Republic of China. It is a good example of a basic TCM gynecology text and covers all of Chinese gynecology, not just menstrual diseases.

The Essence of Liu Feng-wu's Gynecology by Liu Feng-wu, translated by Shuai Xue-zhong & Bob Flaws, Blue Poppy Press, Boulder, CO, 1998. Liu Feng-wu was a famous Chinese gynecologist living in the latter half of this century. This book is a collection of his essays on the practice of Chinese gynecology, a selection of his gynecological case histories, and discussion of some of his personal Chinese herbal formulas. It is a very nice example of a senior Chinese practitioner's personal approach to gynecology.

Fu Qing-zhu's Gynecology by Fu Qing-zhu, translated by Yang Shou-zhong & Liu Da-wei, Blue Poppy Press, Boulder, CO, 1995. Fu Qing-zhu was the greatest gynecologist of ancient China. Living in the late 1700s, Fu Qing-zhu wrote in a very easy to understand, down to earth way. Most of the formulas he created are still used in TCM gynecology today. If one wants to have an historical appreciation for Chinese gynecology, one must read Fu Qing-zhu.

Obstetrics & Gynecology in Chinese Medicine by Giovanni Maciocia, Churchill Livingstone, Edinburgh, 1998. This also a very large clinical manual of all of Chinese gynecology intended for professional practitioners.

For more information on Chinese dietary therapy, see:

The Tao of Healthy, Eating: A Simple Guide to Diet According to Traditional Chinese Medicine by Bob Flaws, Blue Poppy Press, Inc., Boulder, CO, 1997. This book is a layperson's primer on Chinese dietary therapy. It includes detailed sections on the clear, bland diet as well as sections on chronic candidiasis and allergies.

The Book of Jook: Chinese Medicinal Porridges, A Healthy Alternative to the Typical Western Breakfast by Bob Flaws, Blue Poppy Press, Inc., Boulder, CO, 1995. This book is specifically about Chinese medicinal porridges made with very simple combinations of Chinese medicinal herbs.

Chinese Medicinal Wines & Elixirs by Bob Flaws, Blue Poppy Press, Inc., Boulder, CO, 1995. This book is a large collection of simple one, two, and three Chinese medicinal wines which can be made at home.

Chinese Medicinal Teas: Simple, Proven Folk Formulas for Treating Disease & Promoting Health by Zong Xiao-fan & Gary Liscum, Blue Poppy Press, Inc., Boulder, CO, 1997. Like the above two books, this book is about one, two, and three ingredient Chinese medicinal teas which are easy to make and can be used at home as adjuncts to other, professionally prescribed treatments or for the promotion of health and prevention of disease.

The Tao of Nutrition by Maoshing Ni, Union of Tao and Man, Los Angeles, 1989. This book is also a good overview of Chinese dietary therapy written specifically for a Western lay audience.

Harmony Rules: The Chinese Way of Health Through Food by Gary Butt & Frena Bloomfield, Samuel Weiser, Inc., York Beach, ME, 1985. This book tries to make Chinese dietary therapy more easily understandable for Western lay readers. Therefore, its discussion of Chinese dietary therapy is not exactly a standard approach. However, it does include much useful information.

Chinese System of Food Cures: Prevention & Remedies by Henry C. Lu, Sterling Publishing Co., Inc, NY, 1986. This book is somewhat more standard. It includes most of the same information found in *The Tao of Nutrition*. I suggest that you pick one or the other of these.

A Practical English-Chinese Library of Traditional Chinese Medicine: Chinese Medicated Diet ed. by Zhang En-qin, Shanghai

College of Traditional Chinese Medicine Publishing House, Shanghai, 1990. This is a very standard discussion of Chinese dietary therapy written for professional practitioners. However, it is still understandable by nonprofessional readers.

Eating Your Way to Health—Dietotherapy in Traditional Chinese Medicine by Cai Jing-feng, Foreign Languages Press, Beijing, 1988. This is a slim little book which gives the pith of Chinese dietary therapy. The English is not very good, but the information is certainly OK.

For more information on Chinese patent medicines, see:

Clinical Handbook of Chinese Prepared Medicine by Chun-han Zhu, Paradigm Publications, Brookline, MA, 1989. This book is an excellent reference text for Chinese prepared or so-called patent medicines. It uses a professionally accurate, standard translational terminology similar to that used in this book. So readers of this book should feel comfortable with the terminology in that book. It is beautifully designed and laid out and is easy to use. This is most definitely my first choice of books on Chinese patent medicines.

Outline Guide to Chinese Herbal Patent Medicines in Pill Form by Margaret A. Naeser, Boston Chinese Medicine, Boston, 1990. This book contains basically the same information as the preceding title. However, it is a paperback and is more "home-made" through desktop publishing. Therefore, it is a cheaper source of essentially the same information in not so nice a package. It also does not use a professionally accurate, standard translational terminology.

For more information on Chinese herbs and formulas, see:

Chinese Herbal Medicine: Materia Medica by Dan Bensky & Andrew Gamble, Eastland Press, Seattle, 1993. This is the "industry standard" when it comes to descriptions of the basic Chinese materia medica. Under each entry you will find the temperature, flavors, channel-enterings, functions, indications, combinations, dosages, and contraindications of all the most important Chinese medicinals.

Chinese Herbal Medicine: Formulas & Strategies by Dan Bensky & Randall Barolet, Eastland Press, Seattle, 1990. This is the companion volume to the preceding text. It is the industry standard for descriptions of all the main Chinese medicinal formulas. Under each entry, it gives the ingredients and their dosages, functions, indications, dosages and administration of the formula as a whole, and cautions and contraindications of all the most important Chinese formulas.

Oriental Materia Medica: A Concise Guide by Hong-yen Hsu *et al.*, Oriental Healing Arts Institute, Long Beach, CA, 1986. This book is a pharmacopeia similar to Bensky & Gamble's above. The information it contains under each herb is not as complete, but it contains many more medicinals. Therefore, it is the next place to look when Bensky & Gamble do not list a particular Chinese medicinal you are trying to find out about.

A Clinical Guide to Chinese Herbs and Formulae by Chen Song Yu & Li Fei, Churchill Livingstone, Edinburgh, 1993. This book contains basic information on both Chinese herbs as individuals, the main Chinese herbal formulas, and the Chinese herbal treatment of the most common diseases with Chinese herbal medicine. Compared to the above books, this book is essentially meant as a textbook for a *course* on Chinese herbal medicine. In that case, the above books become reference texts for the *practice* of Chinese herbal medicine.

Chinese Herbal Remedies by Albert Y. Leung, Universe Books, NY, 1984. This book is about simple Chinese herbal home remedies.

Legendary Chinese Healing Herbs by Henry C. Lu, Sterling Publishing, Inc., NY, 1991. This book is a fun way to begin learning about Chinese herbal medicine. It is full of interesting and entertaining anecdotes about Chinese medicinal herbs.

For more information on Asian insights into psychology & psychotherapy, see:

The Quiet Therapies: Japanese Pathways to Personal Growth, David K. Reynolds, University of Hawaii Press, Honolulu, 1987. This book is a great little introduction to Japanese forms of psychotherapy based on doing, not analyzing. It also talks about the psychotherapeutic benefits of deep relaxation. David Reynolds has since gone on to author a number of other popular books on Asian insights to psychological health, such as *Playing Ball on Running Water* and *Even in Winter the Ice Doesn't Melt*.

Books with information on Western alternatives for menopausal health

Alternative Medicine Guide to Women's Health, Future Medicine Publishing, Inc., 1998. This guidebook includes other topics besides menopause, but has a variety of interesting information and suggestions on many aspects and stages of women's health.

Menopause Naturally, Preparing for the Second Half of Life, Sadja Greenwood, MD, Volcano Press. A reasonable, sane Western medical description of the various symptoms and possible approaches to treatment and self-help.

A Change for the Better: A Women's Guide Through the Menopause, Patricia Davis and Patricia Davies, Beekman Publishing, Inc. 1994. Good descriptions of the Western medical facts with a variety of ideas for dealing with symptoms.

Natural Woman, Natural Menopause by Marcus Laux and Christine Conrad, Harper Collins, 1998. A naturopathic approach to dealing with menopausal complaints. Lots of vitamins, dietary suggestions, and Western herbs.

Before the Change: Taking Charge of Your Perimenopause, Ann Louise Gittleman, Harper San Francisco, 1998. It's always a good idea to begin preventive therapy before the fact. In Chinese medicine, it is thought that treating after symptoms arise is like digging a well after you are thirsty.

196

16

Chinese Medical Glossary

Chinese medicine is a system unto itself. Its technical terms are uniquely its own and cannot be reduced to the definitions of Western medicine without destroying the very fabric and logic of Chinese medicine. Ultimately, because Chinese medicine was created in the Chinese language, Chinese medicine is best and really only understood in that language. Nevertheless, as Westerners trying to understand Chinese medicine, we must translate the technical terms of Chinese medicine in English words. If some of these technical translations sound at first peculiar and their meaning is not immediately transparent, this is because no equivalent concepts exist in everyday English.

In the past, some Western authors have erroneously translated technical Chinese medical terms using Western medical or at least quasi-scientific words in an attempt to make this system more acceptable to Western audiences. For instance, the words tonify and sedate are commonly seen in the Western Chinese medical literature even though, in the case of sedate, its meaning is 180° opposite to the Chinese understanding of the word *xie*. *Xie* means to drain off something which has pooled and accumulated. That accumulation is seen as something excess which should not be lingering where it is. Because it is accumulating somewhere where it shouldn't, it is impeding and obstructing whatever should be moving to and through that area. The word sedate comes from the Latin word *sedere*, to sit. Therefore, the word sedate means to make something sit still. In English, we get the word sediment from this same root. However, the Chinese *xie* means draining off something which is sitting somewhere erroneously. Therefore, to think that one is going to sedate what is already sitting is a great mistake in understanding the clinical implication and application of this technical term.

Thus, in order, to preserve the integrity of this system while still making it intelligible to English language readers, we have appended the following glossary of Chinese medical technical terms. The terms themselves are based on Nigel Wiseman's *English-Chinese Chinese-English Dictionary of Chinese Medicine* published by the Hunan Science & Technology Press in Changsha, Hunan, People's Republic of China in 1995. Dr. Wiseman is, we believe, the greatest Western scholar in terms of the translation of Chinese medicine into English. As a Chinese reader myself (BF), although I often find Wiseman's terms awkward sounding at first, I also think they convey most accurately the Chinese understanding and logic of these terms.

Acquired essence: Essence manufactured out of the surplus of qi and blood in turn created out of the refined essence of food and drink

Acupoints: Those places on the channels and network vessels where qi and blood tend to collect in denser concentrations, and thus those places where the qi and blood in the channels are especially available for manipulation

Acupuncture: The regulation of qi flow by the stimulation of certain points located on the channels and network vessels achieved mainly by the insertion of fine needles into these points

Aromatherapy: Using various scents and smells to treat and prevent disease

Ascendant hyperactivity of liver yang: Upwardly out of control counterflow of liver yang due to insufficient yin to hold it down in the lower part of the body

Blood: The red colored fluid which flows in the vessels and nourishes and constructs the tissues of the body

Blood stasis: Also called dead blood, malign blood, and dry blood, blood stasis is blood which is no longer moving through the vessels as it should. Instead it is precipitated in the vessels like silt in a river. Like silt, it then obstructs the free flow of the blood in the vessels and also impedes the production of new or fresh blood.

Blood vacuity: Insufficient blood manifesting in diminished nourishment, construction, and moistening of body tissues

Bowels: The hollow yang organs of Chinese medicine

Channels: The main routes for the distribution of qi and blood, but mainly qi

Clear: The pure or clear part of food and drink ingested which is then turned into qi and blood

Counterflow: An erroneous flow of qi, usually upward but sometimes horizontally as well

Dampness: A pathological accumulation of body fluids

Decoction: A method of administering Chinese medicinals by boiling these medicinals in water, removing the dregs, and drinking the resulting medicinal liquid

Depression: Stagnation and lack of movement, as in liver depression qi stagnation

Depressive heat: Pathological heat transformed due to qi depression or stagnation

Drain: To drain off or away some pathological qi or substance from where it is replete or excess

Essence: A stored, very potent form of substance and qi, usually yin when compared to yang qi, but can be transformed into yang qi

Five phase theory: An ancient Chinese system of correspondences dividing up all of reality into five phases of development which then mutually engender and check each other according to definite sequences.

Hydrotherapy: Using various baths and water applications to treat and prevent disease

Life gate fire: Another name for kidney yang or kidney fire, seen as the ultimate source of yang qi in the body.

Magnet therapy: Applying magnets to acupuncture points to treat and prevent disease

Moxibustion: Burning the herb Artemisia Argyium on, over, or near acupuncture points in order to add yang qi, warm cold, or promote the movement of the qi and blood

Network vessels: Small vessels which form a net-like web insuring the flow of qi and blood to all body tissues

Phlegm: A pathological accumulation of phlegm or mucus congealed from dampness or body fluids

Qi: Activity, function, that which moves, transforms, defends, restrains, and warms

Portals: Also called orifices, the openings of the sensory organs and the opening of the heart through which the spirit makes contact with the world outside

Qi mechanism: The process of transforming yin substance controlled and promoted by the qi, largely synonymous with the process of digestion

Qi vacuity: Insufficient qi manifesting in diminished movement, transformation, and function

Repletion: Excess or fullness, almost always pathological

Seven star hammer: A small hammer with needles embedded in its head used to stimulate acupoints without actually inserting needles

Spirit: The accumulation of qi in the heart which manifests as consciousness, sensory awareness, and mental-emotional function

Stagnation: Non-movement of the qi, lack of free flow, constraint

Supplement: To add to or augment, as in supplementing the qi, blood, yin, or yang

Turbid: The yin, impure, turbid part of food and drink which is sent downward to be excreted as waste

Vacuity: Emptiness or insufficiency, typically of qi, blood, yin, or yang

Vacuity cold: Obvious signs and symptoms of cold due to a lack or insufficiency of yang qi

Vacuity heat: Heat due to hyperactive yang in turn due to insufficient controlling yin

Vessels: The main routes for the distribution of qi and blood, but mainly blood

Viscera: The solid yin organs of Chinese medicine

Yang: In the body, function, movement, activity, transformation

Yang vacuity: Insufficient warming and transforming function giving rise to symptoms of cold in the body

Yin: In the body, substance and nourishment

Yin vacuity: Insufficient yin substance necessary to nourish, control, and counterbalance yang activity

Bibliography

Chinese language sources

Bai Ling Fu Ke (Bai-ling's Gynecology), Han Bai-ling, Heilongjiang People's Press, Harbin, 1983

Fu Ke Lin Chuan Jing Hua (The Clinical Efflorescence of Gynecology), Wang Bu-ru & Wang Qi-ming, Sichuan Science & Technology Press, Chengdu, 1989

Fu Ke Yu Chi (The Jade Ruler of Gynecology), Shen Jin-ao, Shanghai Science & Technology Press, Shanghai, 1983

Fu Ke Zheng Zhi (Gynecological Patterns & Treatments), Sun Jiu-ling, Hebei People's Press, 1983

Han Ying Chang Yong Yi Xue Ci Hui (Chinese-English Glossary of Commonly Used Medical Terms), Huang Xiao-kai, People's Health & Hygiene Press, Beijing, 1982

"A Review of the Chinese Medical Literature on Climacteric Syndrome", Yao Shi-an, *Zhong Yi Za Zhi (Journal of Chinese Medicine)*, #2, 1994, p. 112-114

Shang Hai Lao Zhong Yi Jing Yan Xuan Bian (A Selected Compilation of Shanghai Old Doctors' Experiences), Shanghai Science & Technology Press, Shanghai, 1984

"Use of Basal Body Temperature in Pattern Discrimination for Patients with Infertility and Blocked Menstruation", Xia Gui-cheng, *Shang Hai Zhong Yi Yao Za Zhi (Shanghai Journal of Chinese Medicine & Medicinals)*, #10, 1992, p. 18-19

Wan Shi Fu Ren Ke (Master Wan's Gynecology), Wan Quan, aka Wan Mi-zhai, Hubei Science & Technology Press, 1984

203

Yu Xue Zheng Zhi (Static Blood Patterns & Treatments), Zhang Xue-wen, Shanxi Science & Technology Press, Xian, 1986

Zhen Jiu Chu Fang Xue (A Study of Acupuncture & Moxibustion Prescriptions), Wang Dai, Beijing Publishing Co., Beijing, 1990

Zhen Jiu Xue (A Study of Acupuncture & Moxibustion), Qiu Mao-liang *et al.*, Shanghai Science & Technology Press, Shanghai, 1985

Zhen Jiu Yi Xue (An Easy Study of Acupuncture & Moxibustion), Li Shou-xian, People's Health & Hygiene Press, Beijing, 1990

Zhong Guo Min Jian Cao Yao Fang (Chinese Folk Herbal Medicinal Formulas), Liu Guang-rui & Liu Shao-lin, Sichuan Science & Technology Press, Chengdu, 1992

Zhong Guo Zhong Yi Mi Fang Da Quan (A Great Compendium of Chinese National Chinese Medical Secret Formulas), ed. by Hu Zhao-ming, Literary Propagation Publishing Company, Shanghai, 1992

Zhong Yi Bing Yin Bing Ji Xue (A Study of Chinese Medical Disease Causes & Disease Mechanisms), Wu Dun- xu, Shanghai College of TCM Press, Shanghai, 1989

Zhong Yi Fu Ke Zhi Liao Shou Ce (A Handbook of Chinese Medical Gynecological Treatment), Wu Shi-xing & Qi Cheng-lin, Shanxi Science & Technology Press, Xian, 1991

Zhong Yi Hu Li Xue (A Study of Chinese Medical Nursing), Lu Su-ying, People's Health & Hygiene Press, Beijing, 1983

Zhong Yi Lin Chuang Ge Ke (Various Clinical Specialties in Chinese Medicine), Zhang En-qin *et al.*, Shanghai College of TCM Press, Shanghai, 1990

Zhong Yi Ling Yan Fang (Efficacious Chinese Medical Formulas), Lin Binzhi, Science & Technology Propagation Press, Beijing, 1991

Zhong Yi Miao Yong Yu Yang Sheng (Chinese Medicine Wondrous Uses & Nourishing Life), Ni Qi-lan, Liberation Army Press, Beijing, 1993

Zhong Yi Zi Xue Cong Shu (The Chinese Medicine Self-study Series), Vol. 1, "Gynecology", Yang Yi-ya, Hebei Science & Technology Press, Shijiazhuang, 1987

English language sources

A Barefoot Doctor's Manual, revised & enlarged edition, Cloudburst Press, Mayne Isle, 1977

"Bone mass in postmenopausal women after withdrawal of oestrogen/gastragen replacement therapy", C. Christiansen *et al.*, *Lancet*, 1981, Feb. 28; 459-461

""Build Exercise into Your Lifestyle", Anon., *Staying Well Newsletter*, American Chiropractic Assoc., May-June, 1989

Cecil's Textbook of Medicine, 18th Edition, 1988

Chinese-English Terminology of Traditional Chinese Medicine, Shuai Xue-zhong *et al.*, Hunan Science & Technology Press, Changsha, 1983

Chinese-English Manual of Commonly-used Prescriptions in Traditional Chinese Medicine, Ou Ming, ed., Joint Publishing Co., Ltd., Hong Kong, 1989

Chinese Herbal Medicine: Formulas & Strategies, Dan Bensky & Randall Barolet, Eastland Press, Seattle, 1990

Chinese Herbal Medicine: Materia Medica, Dan Bensky & Andrew Gamble, second, revised edition, Eastland Press, Seattle, 1993

A Clinical Guide to Chinese Herbs and Formulae, Cheng Song-yu & Li Fei, Churchill & Livingstone, Edinburgh, 1993

A Clinical Manual of Chinese Herbal Medicine and Acupuncture, Zhou Zhong Ying & Jin Hui De, Churchill Livingstone, Edinburgh, 1997

Chen's History of Chinese Medical Science, Hong-yen Hsu & William G. Preacher, Oriental Healing Arts Institute, Long Beach, CA, 1977

Chinese-English Terminology of Traditional Chinese Medicine, Shuai Xue-zhong, Hunan Science & Technology Press, Changsha, 1981

Chong & Ren Imbalance, Cyclic Management of Menstrual Disorders, Cheng Jing, trans. by C.S. Cheung, Harmonious Sunshine Cultural Center, CA, undated

Clinical Applications of of St. 36, Sp. 6, Co. 4 and 11, and Lu. 7: One Combination of Points Can Treat Many Diseases, Miriam Lee, self-published, Palo Alto, CA, undated

"Comparative effects of oestrogen and a progestogen on bone loss in in postmenopausal women", R. Lindsay *et al.*, *Clinical Science & Molecular Medicine*, 1978; 54:193-195

A Compendium of TCM Patterns & Treatments, Bob Flaws & Daniel Finney, Blue Poppy Press, Boulder, CO, 1996

A Comprehensive Guide to Chinese Herbal Medicine, Chen Ze-lin & Chen Mei-fang, Oriental Healing Arts Institute, Long Beach, CA, 1992

Concise Traditional Chinese Gynecology, Xia Gui-cheng *et al.*, Jiangsu Science & Technology Press, Nanjing, 1988

"Does calcium supplementation prevent postmenopausal bone loss?", B.R. Riis *et al.*, *New England Journal of Medicine*, 1987; 316: 173-177

"Drug-Mineral Interactions", Lois Kramer *et al.*, Fed. Proc, Vol. 43, #4, Abstract, 1281, 1986, p. 375

"Effect of Dietary Caffeine and Sucrose on Urinary Calcium Excretion in Adolescents", P.W. Holling berry *et al.*, Fed. Proc., #45, Abstract, 1986, p. 1286

"Effect of intermittent cyclical etidronate therapy on bone mass and fracture rate in women with postmenopausal osteoporosis", T. Storm *et al.*, *New England Journal of Medicine*, 1990; 322: 1265-1271

English-Chinese Chinese-English Dictionary of Chinese Medicine, Nigel Wiseman, Hunan Science & Technology Press, Changsha, 1995

Estrogen Replacement Therapy, Don R. Gambrell Jr., Essential Medical Information Systems, Inc., Dallas, 1990

"Estrogens in the prevention and treatment of postmenopausal osteoporosis, a review", U.S. Barbel, *American Journal of Medicine*, 1988; 85: 847-850

"Estrogen Treatment of Postmenopausal Women: Benefits and Risks", E.S. Shoemaker, J.P. forney, & P.C. MacDonald, *Journal of the American Medical Association*, #238, Jan. 1977

Free & Easy: Traditional Chinese Gynecology for American Women, Bob Flaws, Blue Poppy Press, Boulder, CO, 1986

Fundamentals of Chinese Acupuncture, Andrew Ellis, Nigel Wiseman & Ken Boss, Paradigm Publications, Brookline, MA, 1988

Fundamentals of Chinese Medicine, Nigel Wiseman & Andrew Ellis, Paradigm Publications, Brookline, MA, 1985

Glossary of Chinese Medical Terms and Acupuncture Points, Nigel Wiseman & Ken Boss, Paradigm Publications, Brookline, MA, 1990

Gynecology & Obstetrics: A Longitudinal Approach, ed. by Thomas R. Moore *et al.,* Churchill Livingstone, NY, 1993

Handbook of Chinese Herbs and Formulas, Him-che Yeung, self-published, LA, 1985

A Handbook of Differential Diagnosis with Key Signs & Symptoms, Therapeutic Principles, and Guiding Prescriptions, Ou-yang Yi, trans. By C.S. Cheung, Harmonious Sunshine Cultural Center, SF, 1987

A Handbook of Menstrual Diseases in Chinese Medicine, Bob Flaws, Blue Poppy Press, Boulder, CO, 1997

Hara Diagnosis: Reflections on the Sea, Kiiko Matsumoto & Stephen Birch, Paradigm Publications, Brookline, MA, 1988

"Is Natural Progesterone the Missing Link in Osteoporosis Prevention & Treatment?", J. R. Lee, *Medical Hypotheses,* #35, 1991, p. 316-318

"Intermittent Cyclic Etidronate Treatment of Postmenopausal Women with Osteoporosis", Nelson B. Watts, *New England Journal of Medicine,* Vol. 323, #2, July 12, 1990

"Mastering Menopause: A Plan of Action for Every Symptom and Side Effect", Gloria MacVeigh, *Prevention Magazine,* Vol. 42, #4, April, 1990, p. 48

"Menopausal Hormone Replacement Therapy with Continuous Daily Oral Micronized Estradiol and Progesterone", Joel T. Hargrove *et al., Gynecology & Obstetrics,* Vol. 73, #4, April 1989, p. 606-612

"Menopause", Gail Sheehy, *Newsweek,* May 25, 1992, p. 79

Menopause Naturally, Preparing for the Second Half of Life, Sadja Greenwood, Volcano Press, Volcano, CA, 1989

Natural Progesterone: The Multiple Roles of a Remarkable Hormone, John Lee, BLL Publishing, Sebastopol, CA, 1993

"Non-hormonal Treatment of Osteoporosis", Allan St. J. Dixon, *British Medical Journal,* Vol. 286, #6370, Mar. 1983

Oriental Materia Medica, A Concise Guide, Hong-yen Hsu, Oriental Healing Arts Institute, Long Beach, CA, 1986

"Osteoporosis of the Slender Smoker: Vertebral Compression Fractures & Loss of Metacarpal Cortex in Relation to Postmenopausal Cigarette Smoking & Lack of Obesity", H.W. Daniell, *Archives of Internal Medicine,* #136, 1976

"Osteoporosis Reversal: The Role of Progesterone", John R. Lee, *International Clinical Nutrition Review,* Vol. 10, #3, July 1990, p. 384-391

Practical Therapeutics of Traditional Chinese Medicine, Yan Wu & Warren Fischer, Paradigm Publications, Brookline, MA, 1997

Practical Traditional Chinese Medicine & Pharmacology: Clinical Experiences, Shang Xian-min *et al.,* New World Press, Beijing, 1990

Practical Traditional Chinese Medicine & Pharmacology: Herbal Formulas, Geng Jun-ying, *et al.,* New World Press, Beijing, 1991

"A Preliminary Discussion of the Bao Gong, Bao Mai, and Bao Luo", Wang Tao-yang, *Blue Poppy Essays, 1988,* Blue Poppy Press, Boulder, CO, 1988

"Preventing Breast Cancer", Julian Whitake, *Health & Healing: Tomorrow's Medicine Today,* Jan. 1994

"Progesterone and Its Relevance for Osteoporosis", Jerilynn C. Prior, *Osteoporosis*, Vol. 2, #2, March 1993

"Progesterone and the Prevention of Osteoporosis", Jerilynn C. Prior *et al.*, *The Canadian Journal of Ob/Gyn & Women's Health Care*, Vol. 3, #4, 1991, p.178-184

"Progesterone as a Bone-trophic Hormone", J.C. Prior, *Endocrine Reviews*, Vol. 11, #2, 1990, p. 386-398

"Reduced Estriol Excretion in Patients with Breast Cancer Prior to Endocrine Therapy", H.M. Lemon, *Journal of the American Medical Association*, 1966, 196:1128-1134

"Report on Menopause", *20'20*, ABC Network TV, Aug. 10, 1990

"Spinal Bone Loss and Ovulatory Disturbances", Jerilynn C. Prior *et al.*, *The New England Journal of Medicine*, Volume 323, #18, November 1, 1990, 1221-1227

"The Case for Progesterone and Osteoporosis", John Lee, *Townsend Letter for Doctors*, Jun. 1993

The English-Chinese Encyclopedia of Practical Traditional Chinese Medicine, Vol. 12: Gynecology, Xuan Jia-sheng, ed., Higher Education Press, Beijing, 1990

The Essential Book of Traditional Chinese Medicine, Vol. 2: Clinical Practice, Liu Yan-chi, trans. by Fang Ting-yu & Chen Lai-di, Columbia University Press, NY, 1988

The Foundations of Chinese Medicine, Giovanni Maciocia, Churchill Livingstone, Edinburgh, 1989

The Genius of China, 3,00 Years of Science, Discoveries, and Invention, Robert Temple, Simon & Schuster, NY, 1989

The Merck Manual, 15th edition, ed. by Robert Berkow, Merck Sharp & Dohme Research Laboratories, Rahway, NJ, 1987

The Nanjing Seminars Transcript, Qiu Mao-lian & Su Xu-ming, The Journal of Chinese Medicine, UK, 1985

The Practice of Chinese Medicine, Giovanni Maciocia, Churchill Livingstone, Edinburgh, 1994

"The Role of the Liver in Menstrual Disorders", (Rona) Wang Ru & Brian May, *The Pacific Journal of Oriental Medicine*, Australia, #77, p. 10-17

The Treatise on the Spleen & Stomach, Li Dong-yuan, trans. by Yang Shou-zhong, Blue Poppy Press, Boulder, CO, 1993

"Uncoupling of bone formation and resorption of combined oestrogen and progestogen therapy in postmenopausal osteoporosis", C. Christiansen *et al.*, *Lancet*, 1985; Oct. 12: 800-801

"Warding Off Breast Cancer", *Newsweek*, Vol. 134, #14, p. 58

The Web That Has No Weaver, Ted Kaptchuk, Congdon & Weed, NY, 1983

"Women's Health Report – Progestrone: Safe antidote for PMS", Lorraine Duskey, *McCall's Magazine*, Oct. 1992, p. 152-156

"Topics in Gynaecology Part One: Menopause", Jane Lyttleton, *Journal of Chinese Medicine* (UK), #33, May, 1990, p. 5

Traditional Medicine in Contemporary China, Nathan Sivin, University of Michigan, Ann Arbor, 1987

Zang Fu: The Organ Systems of Traditional Chinese Medicine, second edition, Jeremy Ross, Churchill Livingstone, Edinburgh, 1985

General Index

A

acquired essence 25, 26, 75, 198
alendronate 160-162
androgens 7, 157
antacids 169
arteries, hardening of the 150

B

back pain 6, 10, 56, 64, 69, 74, 119, 145, 166, 182
bao luo 35, 36, 57
bao mai 35, 36, 57, 209
biofeedback therapy 7
biological age 63
blood, loss of 26, 27
body fat 151
breast cancer 7, 79, 81, 151-153, 209-211
breast disease, fibrocystic 45
breast distention 94, 151
bruising, easy 56

C

caffeine 82, 113-115, 167-169, 207
calcium loss, urinary 168
cardiovascular disease 79, 151
chemotherapy 64
childbearing, excessive 106
cholesterol, high ldl 150
chong mai 36, 37, 41, 42, 57
complexion, pale 69
constipation 59, 60, 67, 74, 136
corticosteroids 169

D

defensive qi 51, 52, 60
diabetes 11, 151, 167

digestive disorders 45
Dilantin 169
drugs, recreational 44, 105

E

edema 47, 64, 69, 151, 155, 158, 180
emotions 17, 23, 27, 30, 39, 46, 47, 54, 80, 94, 113
endocrine system 31
ert 5-7, 125, 149-152, 154-160, 162, 164, 169
estrogen 3-7, 34, 62, 79, 80, 125, 149-154, 159, 162-164, 207
estrogen replacement therapy 5, 6, 62, 125, 149-153, 163, 207
etidronate 160-162, 207, 208
exercise, vigorous 78, 79
eyes, dry 47, 73, 134

F

fat, body 151
fatigue 5, 10, 54-58, 69, 70, 73, 74, 95, 98, 118, 120, 138
fear and anxiety 70
fibrocystic breast disease 45
five phase theory 48, 49, 51, 72, 110, 115, 116, 199
follicle stimulating hormone 3
food, cooked 111
foods, easily digestible 110, 112
foods, frozen 113
foods, spicy 57, 115
frenetic pace 91
frustration 45, 92, 107

G

gallbladder disease 7, 151, 155
genitalia 36, 60

H

healthy menopause 75
heart blood vacuity 54, 56, 71, 121
heart, racing of the 71
heart yin and blood vacuity 71, 121
hormone imbalance 32, 33
hot flashes 5, 6, 46, 48-51, 67, 68, 74, 113, 151, 175, 178
hyperthyroidism 82, 168
hypochondrium 87-88

I, J, K

incontinence 6, 7, 57, 72
insomnia 5, 47, 49, 52-54, 67, 70-72, 74, 102-104, 118, 121, 122, 135, 139-141, 144, 173, 175, 177-180
insulin 11
insulin shock 11
irascibility 47, 68
kidney yang vacuity 43, 58, 61, 62, 69, 97, 119, 132, 138, 182, 183
kidney yin vacuity 43, 58, 67, 132, 137, 182, 183

L

lactose intolerance 169
leukorrhea 72
limbs, heavy 112
listlessness 56
liver blood vacuity 68, 139, 140
liver depression qi stagnation 45, 47-50, 53, 58, 59, 74, 77, 107, 118, 120, 126, 129, 133, 155, 199
liver fire, depressive 47, 53, 99
liver yang hyperactivity, ascendant 68, 99, 132
low back pain 10, 56, 64, 69, 74, 119, 145, 166
lung yin vacuity 58

luteinizing hormone 3

M

marrow bones 116, 117
meditation 93
menopause, artificial 4, 63, 64
menopause, healthy 75
menopause, premature 4, 63, 177
menopausal migraines 68
migraines 68, 151, 155
moxibustion 97, 99, 127, 130, 179-181, 185, 199, 203

N

natural progesterone 153, 162, 164, 207, 208
nausea 7, 56, 58, 70, 151, 155, 160
Nei Jing 23, 41
nicotine 169
night sweats 5, 6, 47, 48, 51, 52, 67, 71, 74, 113, 145, 151

O

obesity 47, 69, 70, 168, 209
oral contraceptives 168
osteoporosis 7, 60, 81, 82, 105, 145, 146, 151, 153, 156, 159, 161-165, 168, 169, 172, 182, 183, 206, 207, 209
overweight 82, 151
overwork 42, 105

P

palms, sweating 73
palpitations 5, 49, 56, 57, 58, 70-72, 74, 118, 119, 122, 135, 139, 140, 145, 173, 175, 179, 180

OTHER BOOKS ON CHINESE MEDICINE AVAILABLE FROM:
BLUE POPPY PRESS

5441 Western, Suite 2, Boulder, CO 80301
For ordering 1-800-487-9296 PH. 303\447-8372 FAX 303\245-8362
Email: info@bluepoppy.com Website: www.bluepoppy.com

ACUPOINT POCKET REFERENCE
by Bob Flaws
ISBN 0-936185-93-7

ACUPUNCTURE & IVF
by Lifang Liang
ISBN 0-891845-24-1

ACUPUNCTURE AND MOXIBUSTION
FORMULAS & TREATMENTS
by Cheng Dan-an, trans. by Wu Ming
ISBN 0-936185-68-6

ACUPUNCTURE PHYSICAL MEDICINE:
An Acupuncture Touchpoint Approach to the
Treatment of Chronic Pain, Fatigue, and
Stress Disorders
by Mark Seem
ISBN 1-891845-13-6

AGING & BLOOD STASIS:
A New Approach to TCM Geriatrics
by Yan De-xin
ISBN 0-936185-63-5
A NEW AMERICAN ACUPUNTURE
By Mark Seem
ISBN 0-936185-44-9

BETTER BREAST HEALTH NATURALLY
with CHINESE MEDICINE
by Honora Lee Wolfe & Bob Flaws
ISBN 0-936185-90-2

THE BOOK OF JOOK:
Chinese Medicinal Porridges
by B. Flaws
ISBN 0-936185-60-0

CHANNEL DIVERGENCES
Deeper Pathways of the Web
by Miki Shima and Charles Chase
ISBN 1-891845-15-2

CHINESE MEDICAL OBSTETRICS
by Bob Flaws
ISBN 1-891845-30-6

CHINESE MEDICAL PALMISTRY:
Your Health in Your Hand
by Zong Xiao-fan & Gary Liscum
ISBN 0-936185-64-3

CHINESE MEDICAL PSYCHIATRY
A Textbook and Clinical Manual
by Bob Flaws and James Lake, MD
ISBN 1-845891-17-9

CHINESE MEDICINAL TEAS:
Simple, Proven, Folk Formulas for
Common Diseases & Promoting Health
by Zong Xiao-fan & Gary Liscum
ISBN 0-936185-76-7

CHINESE MEDICINAL WINES & ELIXIRS
by Bob Flaws
ISBN 0-936185-58-9

CHINESE PEDIATRIC MASSAGE THERAPY:
A Parent's & Practitioner's Guide to the
Prevention & Treatment of Childhood Illness
by Fan Ya-li
ISBN 0-936185-54-6

CHINESE SELF-MASSAGE THERAPY:
The Easy Way to Health
by Fan Ya-li
ISBN 0-936185-74-0

THE CLASSIC OF DIFFICULTIES:
A Translation of the Nan Jing
translation by Bob Flaws
ISBN 1-891845-07-1

CLINICAL NEPHROLOGY
IN CHINESE MEDICINE
by Wei Li & David Frierman,
with Ben Luna & Bob Flaws
ISBN 1-891845-23-3

CONTROLLING DIABETES NATURALLY
WITH CHINESE MEDICINE
by Lynn Kuchinski
ISBN 0-936185-06-3

CURING ARTHRITIS NATURALLY WITH
CHINESE MEDICINE
by Douglas Frank & Bob Flaws
ISBN 0-936185-87-2

CURING DEPRESSION NATURALLY WITH
CHINESE MEDICINE
by Rosa Schnyer & Bob Flaws
ISBN 0-936185-94-5

CURING FIBROMYALGIA NATURALLY
WITH CHINESE MEDICINE
by Bob Flaws
ISBN 1-891845-09-8

CURING HAY FEVER NATURALLY WITH
CHINESE MEDICINE
by Bob Flaws
ISBN 0-936185-91-0

CURING HEADACHES NATURALLY WITH
CHINESE MEDICINE
by Bob Flaws
ISBN 0-936185-95-3

CURING IBS NATURALLY WITH CHINESE
MEDICINE
by Jane Bean Oberski
ISBN 1-891845-11-X

CURING INSOMNIA NATURALLY WITH
CHINESE MEDICINE
by Bob Flaws
ISBN 0-936185-86-4

CURING PMS NATURALLY WITH
CHINESE MEDICINE
by Bob Flaws
ISBN 0-936185-85-6

THE DIVINE FARMER'S MATERIA MEDICA
A Translation of the Shen Nong Ben Cao
translation by Yang Shou-zhong
ISBN 0-936185-96-1

DUI YAO: THE ART OF COMBINING
CHINESE HERBAL MEDICINALS
by Philippe Sionneau
ISBN 0-936185-81-3

ENDOMETRIOSIS, INFERTILITY AND
TRADITIONAL CHINESE MEDICINE:
A Laywoman's Guide
by Bob Flaws
ISBN 0-936185-14-7

THE ESSENCE OF LIU FENG-WU'S
GYNECOLOGY
by Liu Feng-wu, translated by Yang Shou-zhong
ISBN 0-936185-88-0

EXTRA TREATISES BASED ON
INVESTIGATION & INQUIRY:
A Translation of Zhu Dan-xi's Ge Zhi Yu Lun
translation by Yang Shou-zhong
ISBN 0-936185-53-8

FIRE IN THE VALLEY: TCM Diagnosis &
Treatment of Vaginal Diseases
by Bob Flaws
ISBN 0-936185-25-2

FU QING-ZHU'S GYNECOLOGY
trans. by Yang Shou-zhong and Liu Da-wei
ISBN 0-936185-35-X

FULFILLING THE ESSENCE:
A Handbook of Traditional & Contemporary
Treatments for Female Infertility
by Bob Flaws
ISBN 0-936185-48-1

GOLDEN NEEDLE WANG LE-TING: A 20th
Century Master's Approach to Acupuncture
by Yu Hui-chan and Han Fu-ru, trans. by Shuai
Xue-zhong
ISBN 0-936185-789-3

A GUIDE TO GYNECOLOGY
by Ye Heng-yin,
trans. by Bob Flaws and Shuai Xue-zhong
ISBN 1-891845-19-5

A HANDBOOK OF TCM PATTERNS
& TREATMENTS
by Bob Flaws & Daniel Finney
ISBN 0-936185-70-8

A HANDBOOK OF TRADITIONAL
CHINESE DERMATOLOGY
by Liang Jian-hui, trans. by Zhang Ting-liang &
Bob Flaws
ISBN 0-936185-07-4

A HANDBOOK OF TRADITIONAL
CHINESE GYNECOLOGY

by Zhejiang College of TCM, trans. by Zhang
Ting-liang & Bob Flaws
ISBN 0-936185-06-6 (4th edit.)

A HANDBOOK OF CHINESE HEMATOLOGY
by Simon Becker
ISBN 1-891845-16-0

A HANDBOOK OF MENSTRUAL DISEASES
IN CHINESE MEDICINE
by Bob Flaws
ISBN 0-936185-82-1

A HANDBOOK of TCM PEDIATRICS
by Bob Flaws
ISBN 0-936185-72-4

THE HEART & ESSENCE OF DAN-XI'S
METHODS OF TREATMENT
by Xu Dan-xi, trans. by Yang Shou-zhong
ISBN 0-926185-49-X

HERB TOXICITIES & DRUG INTERACTIONS:
A Formula Approach
by Fred Jennes with Bob Flaws
ISBN 1-891845-26-8

IMPERIAL SECRETS OF HEALTH
& LONGEVITY
by Bob Flaws
ISBN 0-936185-51-1

INSIGHTS OF A SENIOR ACUPUNCTURIST
by Miriam Lee
ISBN 0-936185-33-3

INTRODUCTION TO THE USE OF
PROCESSED CHINESE MEDICINALS
by Philippe Sionneau
ISBN 0-936185-62-7

KEEPING YOUR CHILD HEALTHY WITH
CHINESE MEDICINE
by Bob Flaws
ISBN 0-936185-71-6

THE LAKESIDE MASTER'S STUDY
OF THE PULSE
by Li Shi-zhen, trans. by Bob Flaws
ISBN 1-891845-01-2

MASTER HUA'S CLASSIC OF THE
CENTRAL VISCERA
by Hua Tuo, trans. by Yang Shou-zhong
ISBN 0-936185-43-0

MASTER TONG'S ACUPUNCTURE
by Miriam Lee
ISBN 0-926185-37-6

THE MEDICAL I CHING: Oracle of the
Healer Within
by Miki Shima
ISBN 0-936185-38-4

MANAGING MENOPAUSE NATURALLY
with Chinese Medicine
by Honora Lee Wolfe
ISBN 0-936185-98-8

NCCAOM BIO-MEDICINE TEST PREP BOOK:
EXAM PREPARATION & STUDY GUIDE
by Zhong Bai-song
ISBN 978-1-891845-34-9

POINTS FOR PROFIT: The Essential Guide
to Practice Success for Acupuncturists
by Honora Wolfe, Eric Strand & Marilyn Allen
ISBN 1-891845-25-X

THE PULSE CLASSIC:
A Translation of the Mai Jing
by Wang Shu-he, trans. by Yang Shou-zhong
ISBN 0-936185-75-9

SHAOLIN SECRET FORMULAS for
Treatment of External Injuries
by De Chan, trans. by Zhang Ting-liang &
Bob Flaws
ISBN 0-936185-08-2

STATEMENTS OF FACT IN TRADITIONAL
CHINESE MEDICINE
by Bob Flaws
ISBN 0-936185-52-X

STICKING TO THE POINT 1:
A Rational Methodology for the Step by
Step Formulation & Administration of
an Acupuncture Treatment
by Bob Flaws
ISBN 0-936185-17-1

STICKING TO THE POINT 2:
A Study of Acupuncture & Moxibustion
Formulas and Strategies
by Bob Flaws
ISBN 0-936185-97-X

A STUDY OF DAOIST ACUPUNCTURE &
MOXIBUSTION
by Liu Zheng-cai
ISBN 1-891845-08-X

THE SUCCESSFUL CHINESE HERBALIST
by Bob Flaws and Honora Lee Wolfe
ISBN 1-891845-29-2

THE SYSTEMATIC CLASSIC OF
ACUPUNCTURE & MOXIBUSTION
A translation of the Jia Yi Jing
by Huang-fu Mi, trans. by Yang Shou-zhong &
Charles Chace
ISBN 0-936185-29-5

THE TAO OF HEALTHY EATING
ACCORDING TO CHINESE MEDICINE
by Bob Flaws
ISBN 0-936185-92-9